The
Uses of Psychiatry
in
Smaller General Hospitals

The
Uses of Psychiatry
in
Smaller General Hospitals

Raymond M. Glasscote, M.A.
CHIEF, JOINT INFORMATION SERVICE

Jon E. Gudeman, M.D.
ASSOCIATE PROFESSOR OF PSYCHIATRY
HARVARD MEDICAL SCHOOL

Allan Beigel, M.D.
PROFESSOR OF PSYCHIATRY
UNIVERSITY OF ARIZONA
COLLEGE OF MEDICINE

A publication of

The Joint Information Service
of the American Psychiatric Association
and the National Mental Health Association

Library of Congress Cataloging in Publication Data

Glasscote, Raymond M.
  The uses of psychiatry in smaller general hospitals.

  1. Psychiatric hospitals—United States. I. Gudeman,
Jon E., 1936–   II. Beigel, Allan. III. Title.
[DNLM: 1. Hospitals, General—United States.
2. Psychiatry. 3. Psychiatric department, Hospital.
WM 27 AA1 G5u]
RC439.G476 1982   362.2′1   82-22719
ISBN 0-89042-108-0 (pbk.)

Printed in the U.S.A.

ACKNOWLEDGEMENT

This book results from an investigation carried out with major support from the van Amerigen Foundation.

CONTENTS

PART I

Background, Overview, and Summary

Background, Overview, and Summary

O F THE NUMEROUS components of psychiatric and mental health services which have become available in the past several decades, the immense development of psychiatric inpatient services in community general hospitals is certainly among the least noticed and documented. It has been almost two decades since the number of admissions per year to psychiatric units of community general hospitals *surpassed* the number of admissions to state hospitals. It is not unfair to say that community general hospital psychiatric units for some considerable years have been doing a major part of the inpatient treatment of psychiatric cases while getting a minor part of the attention.

*   *   *

Enthusiasts of psychiatric services in community general hospitals have credited such units, of which there are by 1982 several hundred, with having reduced over a period of years the typical census of the state hospitals by something more than three-quarters. This well-intentioned attribution is only partially correct. It is true that by the early 1950's the census, at a given time, of the state hospitals was more than half a million pa-

3

tients, that the census had risen steadily for decades (except for a two-year period during World War II), and that by 1956 it had reached 556,000. But in the following year, the census fell slightly, and it continued to fall, at an ever-increasing rate, so that by 1980 the typical census of state hospitals was only 132,000.

The availability of inpatient psychiatric treatment in community general hospitals certainly was one major factor in this remarkable emptying out of the state mental hospitals. But it was by no means the only factor. It was at approximately the middle of the decade of the 1950's that newly available ''antipsychotic'' medications began to be broadly used in mental hospitals. These drugs served in the majority of schizophrenics to prevent hallucinations and delusions and in other ways obviate those behaviors of psychotic patients which had kept them hospitalized—in part because of their limited ability to function in communities and in part because of the fear generated by their unusual behaviors. Very shortly afterward, the ''anti-depressant'' medications became available, and these served, in the majority of severely depressed patients, to terminate the depression. Consequently, the advent of previously unavailable pharmaceuticals played a major part in the reduction of census of the state mental hospitals.

An increase in access to *outpatient* treatment also was a factor. The numbers of psychiatrists completing training during the 1950's and on into and through the following decade was such that in many communities where outpatient psychiatric treatment had been unavailable—resulting, thus, in many patients being sent to some distant state mental hospital—the situation changed. Psychiatrists in office practice increased in number in the cities and began increasingly to be available in the towns. To some unmeasured and at this point unknowable extent, the greater availability of outpatient psychiatric practitioners also surely accelerated the decline in the census of public mental hospitals.

The availability of private *health insurance* coverage to reimburse the costs of treatment of hospitalization for psychiatric reasons came relatively late, and slowly and cautiously, but early experience was "gratifying" in the sense that the volume of claims and the volume of dollars paid out for inpatient care were not considered prohibitive. Consequently, the inclusion of psychiatric services within such health insurance policies grew, and in time became a very large consideration in the decision of community general hospitals to develop psychiatric wards. Accordingly, persons who had gone, or been taken, to state hospitals because they could not have afforded to pay for care in a community general hospital were now able to do so, and thereby a further inducement to the development and growth of general hospital psychiatry emerged.

There were various other components of the startling decline in population of state mental hospitals, but we will conclude by taking note of changes in policies and practices within those hospitals, in part as the result of court rulings and in part because of changing attitudes regarding civil rights of "proposed" patients, in the processes of commitment, and in similar legal aspects that came to be major considerations. To simplify, just as it had once been a relatively simple matter to arrange for the admission of a person to a state mental hospital, with time it became increasingly difficult.

*   *   *

Thus, several developments and influences were all involved in the decline in state mental hospital populations over the years. And certainly quite major among these has been the increasing availability of, and the increasingly available means to pay for, treatment in psychiatric units of community general hospitals. That the significance of these treatment resources was not being fully acknowledged became a concern of the Joint Information Service, which began in the 1960's to study community general hospital psychiatric services. A survey which it carried out in 1964 and published in 1965 established for the first time that psychiatric admissions to community general hospitals had come to exceed in number the admissions to the several hundred state and county mental hospitals around the country.

This particular study showed that the "growth phase" of community general hospital services began almost immediately after the end of World War II; that the growth had continued at an ever-accelerating rate; and that by 1963 more than half of "large" general hospitals had such units—specifically, 52 percent of hospitals having between 400 and 500 beds and 75 percent of hospitals having 500 and more beds. A subsequent study showed that in the ensuing decade the rate of establishing psychiatric units in community general hospitals had not only held up but had continued to increase.

*   *   *

Going back to the earliest days of hospitals, and because of actual and imagined differences between psychiatric patients and medical and surgical patients, it was supposed, with extremely rare exceptions, that the two groups should not be served within the same facility. For the most part, even the earliest established psychiatric inpatient units at medical schools were housed unto themselves in separate buildings. Suffice it to say that by the time the United States entered World War II, in 1941, there were, according to the best data available, no more than forty general hospitals that had psychiatric units, wards, wings, or even separate buildings for psychiatric patients on their grounds.

But almost immediately after World War II, general hospitals began, at first in small numbers but soon at an ever-increasing rate, to set up psychiatric units, wards, or wings. One can no more than speculate the various reasons for so dramatic a change, beginning as it did years before the new pharmaceuticals and the broadening of psychiatric benefits in health insurance policies. But clearly a major factor was the experience of military psychiatry during World War II, when it was widely observed that, by and large, many of the soldiers who became emotionally impaired or who became dysfunctional for evident emotional reasons, and who were promptly treated at the site of "breakdown" and soon returned to duty, had a considerably better ultimate outcome than those emotionally disabled troops who were evacuated to distant military hospitals.

In any event, for a community general hospital to have a psychiatric unit ceased, within a decade after the war, to be a rarity, and became fairly common. The first Joint Information Service survey of psychiatric units in general hospitals found that by 1942 there were only 39 such units whereas eight years later, by the end of 1950, the number had nearly doubled, to 73. By the end of 1958, it had more than redoubled, to 164. A subsequent JIS survey found that the trend continued and that by the end of 1971 there were at least 726 community general hospitals that had psychiatric inpatient units.

* * *

What was notable in both surveys was the likelihood that a community general hospital would have a psychiatric unit was clearly related to its total bed size. Specifically:

Total beds in hospital	No. of hospitals in U.S. of this bed size, 1971	Percent reporting that the hospital had a psychiatric unit	
		1963 survey	1971 survey
500 and more	230	75	80
400–499	188	52	60
300–399	351	29	49
200–299	578	16	24
100–199	1,222	5	10
Less than 100	3,092	1	1

As can be seen, in the eight years between the two surveys the percentage of hospitals reporting a psychiatric unit had increased in all but the smallest of the bed-size categories which we used.

Even so, as of 1971 only ten percent of the hospitals having from one hundred to two hundred beds had such a unit, and only one percent of the great many more hospitals having fewer than a hundred beds; hospitals of such small total size comprised, specifically, more than three-quarters of all the country's community general hospitals (76.2 percent), and those hospitals having fewer than one hundred beds accounted for more than half (54.6 percent).

*　　*　　*

We now shift focus.

In the early 1950's, by which time there were more than half a million patients, at a given time, in the country's state (and a few county) mental hospitals, the then president of the American Psychiatric Association, speaking at a meeting of that organization's Hospital and Community Psychiatry Institute (then known as the Mental Hospital Institute) called for the establishment of a temporary, national, high-level commission to study the dimensions of the problems of mental illness and of the adequacy of existing treatment resources to deal with it, and to formulate a plan whereby to improve and expand treatment resources to the extent found to be needed.

Congress soon thereafter chartered the Joint Commission on Mental Illness and Health, which was authorized and funded to spend five years carrying out its charge and to submit its report to the Congress. It did so in December 1960.

The report recommended expanded activity in research—mainly basic research with emphasis on the *causes* of mental illnesses—and for federal support in one form or another for higher education (*all* higher education, not just that specific to the mental health field). It also recommended that efforts be made to operate existing mental hospitals as open facilities "as part of an integrated community service with emphasis on outpatient and aftercare facilities as well as inpatient services." It recommended that research programs be established "in selected state mental hospitals and community mental health programs." It recommended that both professional and "subprofessional" training be "establish[ed] in selected state mental hospitals and community programs."

It made a number of other recommendations, in several areas. Concerning treatment services, it particularly addressed the general hospital:

> No community general hospital should be regarded as rendering a complete service unless it accepts mental patients for short-term hospitalization and therefore provides a psychiatric unit or psychiatric beds. Every community general hospital of 100 or more beds should make this provision. . . . It is the consensus of the Mental Health Study that definitive care for patients with major mental ill-

ness should be given if possible, or for as long as possible, in a psychiatric unit of a general hospital. . . . *

The Commission's report was studied by a Cabinet-level group appointed by then-President John F. Kennedy. On the basis of that group's specific legislative recommendations, Kennedy in 1963 sent to the Congress a special message concerning mental illness and health. Foremost among the recommendations of that message was that Congress authorize and fund a facility which Kennedy referred to as the Community Mental Health Center— and which he referred to as a "bold, new approach." At that point in time, the community mental health center had not been defined, nor was it to be defined until after Congress passed legislation authorizing such a national program. When definition did come, it came from within what was then the Department of Health, Education, and Welfare.

The community mental health center as HEW defined it would provide, if it were to meet HEW's definition of "comprehensive," some eleven specific services. And for a proposed center to qualify at all for the authorized federal funds to provide partial financial support, it would be required to provide not less than five stipulated services from among these eleven.

Consequently, it is neither unfair nor misleading to say that the community mental health center program, as it came into being, was a far cry from anything recommended by the Joint Commission on Mental Illness and Health. The HEW regulations for the "centers program" served, among other things, to rule out of consideration for partial federal support any smaller community general hospital that might wish to apply for these

---

*Joint Commission on Mental Illness and Health, *Action for Mental Health: Final Report of the Joint Commission on Mental Illness and Health,* Basic Books, 1961.

funds to help in starting an inpatient psychiatric service but which felt itself unable or disinclined to undertake to establish at one and the same time a program of not less than five stipulated psychiatric services.

It seems quite likely that these factors account to a considerable extent for the fact that by 1982 only a small minority of the hospitals having fewer than 200 beds have an inpatient psychiatric unit.

*   *   *

Although (a) the Joint Commission's report at one point stated that all community general hospitals should have psychiatric beds, and at another that all such hospitals having one hundred or more beds should have a psychiatric *unit,* and (b) by 1982 only a small fraction of the former group and a minuscule fraction of the latter group do in fact have such services and units, these are not the reasons underlying this present study.

When the Joint Information Service undertook its first, and mainly statistical, survey of general hospital psychiatric units, its staff was surprised to learn that so large a number of the community general hospitals in this country are so small in size—with only 1,347 of 5,661 having as many as two hundred beds. We are not concerned, in this present study, with the likelihood that the thousand or so largest hospitals may well have among them far more total beds than do the several thousand smaller hospitals. Our concern, which began years ago and eventuated in this study, stems from our awareness that a great many of the smaller hospitals are located in towns and villages that are a considerable distance from any other hospital that does provide inpatient psychiatric service.

We have encountered in the research that was necessary to this present study only one publication wherein the authors question whether it is of any advantage or benefit for psychiatric patients to have hospital facilities close at hand. One need hardly say that the authors who raise that question have no data indicating that it is not; and contrariwise we have no data indicating that it is. Such data have not been available from comparative studies. But we have taken it as a given, and we believe that the substantial majority of people do, that health services should be readily accessible and that there are reasonable grounds on which to maintain that readily accessible health services are, with rare and idiosyncratic exceptions, both advantageous to most patients, and an obligation, in the same sense that readily available schools, fire departments, and police services are, with rare exceptions, considered necessary. We have subscribed to the viewpoint that a person in need of inpatient psychiatric treatment should not find it necessary to travel (or be transported) some fifty miles or more in order to obtain it.

*   *   *

It was our intention, consequently, in deciding to undertake this study, to develop information that might eventuate in causing some of the many small hospitals not having psychiatric units to consider whether it might be appropriate for them to investigate and consider the matter. The thrust of this present study was thus quite simple: (a) to identify all of that small number of small general hospitals that had already developed psychiatric units; (b) to send each of them a questionnaire asking for limited but highly intentional information about their units; (c) from those responses to select not more than ten seeming to be both evidently successful and differing from each other as much as possible in such matters as number of beds for psychiatry, geographic location and other demographic aspects, staffing, and the like; (d) to arrange with those hospitals for the senior author and one (in each instance) of the other two authors to visit the facility and during that visit to have interviews with a broad variety of staff, patients, the hospital administrator, attending staff physicians including and additional to psychiatrists, pertinent staff from community agencies that are germane to the successful operation of the psychiatric unit, and others, as time allowed; (e) assuming that at least the majority of the ten visited did, in fact, appear to be successful and of good quality, to prepare a publication consisting mainly of detailed descriptions of the individual facilities visited.

For our first step in identifying those smaller hospitals having psychiatric units, we had available directories and guides to hospitals prepared and issued by three different sources. Because in prior studies of other aspects of treatment services we had found that the error rate was quite high in some such directories, we consequently after having compiled all of the names and addresses sent an "identifying questionnaire" to the administrator of each such hospital listed, asking three questions only: the total number of beds in his hospital; whether the hospital in fact had a separate psychiatric unit "as contrasted with admitting patients with psychiatric diagnoses to general medical and surgical beds"; and, if there was a separate psychiatric unit, the name of the chief of service.

We suspected in advance that one of the directories might contain a high rate of error; that is, would have listed many small hospitals as having separate psychiatric units when in fact they did not. Our suspicion proved warranted. Thirty-four of the responding hospitals were outside the scope of this study, in most cases because they did not in fact have a separate psychiatric unit and in some cases because the indicated total bed size of the hospital was considerably larger than the specifications for this study. In addition three hospitals had closed down, two had closed down their psychiatric units, and two were general hospitals in each case serving only a particular prison. (Our survey was by intention limited to *community* general hospitals serving the general public, thereby excluding those that serve only a limited or specialized clientele—as, for example, general hospitals within prisons, mental hospitals, or other institutions, or those serving only an "entitled" clientele, such as the Veterans Administration hospitals.)

Because we felt from the outset that we might not be able to identify ten hospitals seemingly suitable to visit from among so small a number indicated to have both a psychiatric unit and a total bed count of less than one hundred, we intentionally included those hospitals indicated to have up to 150 beds; and, as it turned out, several of those selected for inclusion in this report did have more than one hundred beds (but fewer than 150). Of the "in scope" responses from the hospital administrators, there were 13 hospitals that had fewer than one hundred beds, two that had exactly one hundred beds, and 19 that had between 101 and 149 beds.

*   *   *

Having thus obtained the name of the chief of service for the psychiatric units, we wrote to each as follows:

Dear Doctor ——————— :

The administrator of your hospital has advised us that it has a separate psychiatric section, unit, or ward and that you are chief of service.

As you probably know, the great majority of "larger" hospitals do have such units. However, "smaller" hospitals, those with fewer than 150 beds, rarely do—in fact, something less than three percent—and these smaller hospitals account for two-thirds or more of all general hospitals in the country.

We are undertaking a study of those few small hospitals that do have psychiatric units, in the hope that we can encourage others to develop them. In this regard, we would greatly appreciate your doing two things for us:

(1) Send one copy each of any brochures, annual reports, or any other kind of descriptive material particular to the psychiatric unit;

(2) Answer the questions on the enclosed sheet.

Because of the special purpose and goal of this study, we hope very much that you can give us this assistance.

Thank you in advance for your help.

Twenty-three of the 34 replied. Two of these told us that definite plans had already been made, in one case to close the psychiatric unit, in the other to close the hospital. From the remaining 21 responses, and on the basis of their answers to the survey form we sent them and the supporting materials which they sent us, and mindful of our desire for variety among them, ten were selected for the field visits, and all ten agreed for us to come.

The survey form then sent to the chiefs of psychiatry asked the following:

1. The year the psychiatric unit began operation
2. Whether federal, state, or local grants, contracts, or other financial support had helped to finance establishing the psychiatric unit
3. Whether, after opening, the unit had received any federal, state, or local grants, contracts, or other financial support
4. The number of beds in the psychiatric unit

5. The average percent of occupancy during the most recent full year for which statistics were available
6. Whether any portion of the psychiatric unit was designated for and/or limited to children, adolescents, geriatric patients, alcoholism patients, drug abuse patients, or any other special categories
7. Whether the unit accepted Medicaid and Medicare patients
8. Whether the psychiatric unit was of public, nonprofit, or private ownership or control
9. What categories of physicians were authorized to admit to the unit
10. What categories of physicians were authorized to attend patients after their admissions
11. The average length of stay
12. The number of *individuals* admitted to the unit during the latest full year for which statistics were available
13. The number of staff, in full-time equivalents or fractions thereof, in ten categories (for example, nurses, social workers)
14. The distance to the nearest state hospital
15. Whether any categories of patients were excluded because of diagnosis, age, or any other basis

*   *   *

Because of other commitments of the authors, it was necessary to spread the visits, and consequently they were made at various times in 1979, the last near the end of that year. Certainly the units differed to a significant degree and in significant ways, as we had hoped they would. On the basis of observing each service and of interviewing, in almost all cases individually, approximately 25 persons at each place visited, it was our conclusion that nine of them were successful and useful operations that were being conducted in appropriate and skillful ways, with well-trained staff and good leadership. In the major section of this report, which describes the programs individually, three of the ten visited are not included. Two, although they were felt to be of superior quality, are excluded because they were so similar in a number of ways to other programs already visited that we felt to include detailed descriptions of them would make this volume repetitious. These were the Woodland Hospital, in Woodland, California, about 30 miles from Sacramento, and St. John's Hospital, in Longview, Washington, about 50 miles north of Portland, Oregon. The tenth facility was not included in this report because it became evident during our visit that it was ineptly administered, chaotic, unnecessarily expensive, and providing inappropriate treatment services. (Were it not for the fact that the unit had a mission to take care of sick people, then it would be no exaggeration to say that it was a farce.)

*   *   *

Conceivably by this point in time a great many persons who would have a say in determining whether a particular smaller general hospital should start a psychiatric unit will have had some personal exposure to one, either in their work, by visiting a friend or relative hospitalized in one, or by having themselves been a patient therein. Consequently, we think the specific requirements for and components of such a service can be briefly stated.

(1) *Bed size.* In general, psychiatric units in general hospitals have about the same number of beds as do most other specialized services. It was frequently asserted, in earlier years, that general hospital psychiatric units should have at least twenty beds in order to be able to afford the variety of personnel thought essential for proper staffing. It appears that increasingly this concept of "minimum size" has lost its hold, and it was interesting to us that two of the units we most appreciated among these ten visited had accommodations for only ten patients. But even

among the small number of hospitals we visited the size of the psychiatric unit varied, so that the largest of them had more than twice the capacity of the smallest. There seems to be persuasive evidence that a unit even as small as ten beds can be appropriately staffed and can afford to provide the appropriate services, activities, and amenities.

(2) *Staffing*. In our preliminary "prestudy" investigations, we learned of only one inpatient service whose director was not a physician. It appears that, given longstanding hospital practice and legal considerations, for the indefinite future the chief of a medical service shall be required to be a physician. Of the ten services that we visited, all were headed by physicians, in every case except one by a psychiatrist; the one exception was the hospital in Longview, Washington, where there was no chief of service but rather a committee, and the head of that committee was a general practice physician who had long practiced in that community and was highly regarded by his fellow physicians.

The nursing staff, even of a very small unit, should have in charge a nurse who has been trained in and/or has extensive experience working with psychiatric patients. This was the case in all of the facilities we visited. In all of the seven later described, this charge nurse was supported by an appropriate number of registered nurses and licensed practical nurses who either had prior experience in working with psychiatric patients or had, under supervision of good quality, the necessary experience gained on the job.

The other staff personnel in the facilities visited—social workers, psychologists, occupational and recreational therapists, and occasionally others—are indicated in the individual descriptions. Suffice it to say that the numbers and the varieties differed considerably. Overall, the ratio of staff to patients seemed in every case adequate, but the presence of various categories of specialized personnel differed in terms of the priorities and concepts of the service, and with the availability and recruitability to and in places which, in some instances, were fairly remote, and also with particular needs and characteristics of the community being served.

(3) *Restrictions on admissions.* It has been charged—frequently, in earlier years—that general hospital psychiatric units and state mental hospitals served very different clienteles, by which was meant, among other things, that the general hospitals declined to admit the "difficult" patients—the patients who posed problems in their behavior and lack of willingness to "cooperate." Given the now considerably larger number of admissions to general hospital psychiatric units than to state mental hospitals, the "differentness" formerly ascribed must surely somehow have diminished greatly. And given the many hundreds of general hospitals that for some years have had psychiatric units, the ascribed selectiveness of their admission policies has surely ameliorated. (In this present study, only two hospitals had any rooms that could be rendered "secure" in the sense of being the old-time locked ward, and it was rarely necessary at either hospital to activate the security features; when this was done, some member of the nursing staff, by regulation, had to look in on the patient each half hour. Restraint devices, such as camisoles ["straitjackets"] were in most cases not available and where available almost never used.)

And rarely were patients transferred from these units to other and "more secure" hospitals. Consequently, there were very few patients excluded on the grounds of their "unmanageable" behavior, either at time of presentation for evaluation, or subsequently. At none of these ten services, however, were children admitted, and all had a stipulated lower age limit, usually

16. And there were few admissions of deteriorated, forgetful older patients of the kind that usually, as a matter of course, in most communities, are denoted to be "senile" and are presented directly to nursing homes on the doing of their primary care physician in collaboration with the patient's relatives.

(4) *Security.* Today, and for many years past, the practice of locking off the psychiatric unit has varied, and some of the best-reputed community general hospital units the authors have visited were kept locked at all times. Among the ten included in this study, only one was consistently locked. We were told by various of this hospital's staff that this was done because the patients preferred to be in a locked ward, the premise being one of excluding from entry unauthorized persons rather than the need to prohibit the exit of patients. We suspected, however, that it was germane, in this unit, alone among the ten, that at most times a considerable number of patients were adolescents, many of them rebellious against their parents and a number of other things. In any case, none of the patients we interviewed at this hospital gave any indication that they minded being on a locked ward.

Other of the units we visited were locked "selectively." Unless there were an evidently "escape-inclined" patient, the entry way to the psychiatric service was unlocked. If there were an evidently elope-prone patient, the entryway was locked.

The majority of the ten units, however, were entirely open, in the sense that there were no restricting or restraining features of any kind pertaining to entry into or exit from the unit. This practice had rarely caused any problem at all with other services of the hospital, and such problems as had occurred had been occasional and minor—as, for instance, when a confused patient wandered off the ward and into one of the medical or surgical wards or into the common areas of the hospital; the response, when this did happen, was coolheaded.

There were, regularly, stipulations about what individual ones of the psychiatric patients might do. In most units, there were "privilege levels," pertaining for the most part to the patient's freedom to leave the ward to go to the hospital's canteen or gift shop, to take walks on the grounds, and to use the telephone. From "zero" level, at which the patient was not permitted to leave the ward under any circumstances, one moves to "level one," meaning that the patient may leave the ward only if accompanied by a staff member, then "level two," under which patients may leave when accompanied by other patients at the same or higher privilege level, and "level three," which customarily meant "full" privileges, specifically the right of the patient to leave the building with staff permission, unaccompanied, although usually not to leave the hospital grounds.

(5) *Activities*. The psychiatric unit differs from all others in community general hospitals in that it is intended for most patients to limit their hours in bed to necessary nighttime sleep, and the rest of the time to be up and about—reading, watching television, conversing with other patients, engaging in group meetings, scheduled crafts, and exercise classes; and for all patients whose condition permits, there were activities outside the hospital at reasonable intervals, for example, walks accompanied by a staff member, visits to a shopping center, or a trip to the movies or some special event such as an exhibit or fair. Several useful purposes are served by these various activities denoted as "activity therapy" and "occupational therapy." They encourage good physical health and the capacity to engage and participate in the ordinary events of daily living, serving not only to reduce boredom and excessive dwelling on one's symptoms and cir-

cumstances, but also to learn new skills and hobbies and how to spend leisure time appropriately.

All of the hospitals visited in this study were providing an adequate amount and variety of such activities, in some cases having specially trained activities and crafts therapists—usually part-time and being shared with other services in the hospital—while in other cases making do with nurses, aides, or whatever other staff members were interested, available, and appropriate.

Perhaps because the average stay in these units was a matter of days, up to no more than two to three weeks, we heard little mention of patients being given passes that would allow them to leave the hospital and stay overnight or spend a weekend with family and significant others.

The considerable majority of patients were permitted to receive visitors, this privilege being withheld only for substantial reason, and visiting hours were, in general, liberal.

(6) *Therapy*. In addition to the ward activities, patients participated in, and were often *required* to participate in, various types of therapy on the units. All patients were under medical care and received visits from their physicians, who in most units and for most patients were psychiatrists. There were various forms of therapeutic counseling provided by psychiatrists, nurses, sometimes social workers, and occasionally psychologists. In form this ranged from task-oriented groups to more structured interpersonal groups. Some counseling seemed quite didactic, some was non-directive, and some was in open-ended groups.

Social workers frequently met with family members, in family or conjoint therapy. Frequently the social worker on the unit helped in arranging for and planning the hospital care.

To varying extents a therapeutic interdisciplinary team was

used—although not at all in some units. If there was one thing that especially stood out, it was the overall *medical* treatment, with therapeutic procedures, medications, and germane other physical treatment under the direction of the psychiatrist.

(7) *The administrators of the hospitals*. We asked in each case to be scheduled for an interview with the administrator. These individuals ranged in background from those with graduate degrees in hospital administration to those who had learned on the job, working their way up the career ladder. All expressed their support of the psychiatric unit and all understood that the unit both broadened the conception of a "medical center" and helped financially in that the psychiatric units ran relatively high occupancy rates. None identified any special problem specific to a psychiatric unit that had not been readily solved.

(8) *Internal relationships*. There was in every one of the hospitals a sense of separateness and difference concerning the psychiatric unit. With one exception, nursing staff from the psychiatric unit did not fill in when there was an unusual shortage of nurses on other services, nor did those from other services fill in on psychiatry. But it appeared that any sense of "estrangement" probably was no greater than in the case of other special-purpose units such as intensive care, pediatrics, and obstetrics; the stigma historically attributed to psychiatric patients was not in evidence.

The Pros and Cons of Starting a Psychiatric Unit

WHILE THE GROWTH through the years of psychiatric units in community general hospitals of large size is impressive, the recommendation of the original Joint Commission on Mental Illness and Health that all general hospitals should have psychiatry beds and that no general hospital with one hundred or more beds should be considered to provide a sufficiently comprehensive service without a psychiatric unit is, by 1982, far from met. As we earlier saw, only a small percentage of hospitals having two hundred or fewer beds have such units, and such units are still scarcer in that large number of hospitals having fewer than one hundred beds.

We believe that the chapters that follow indicate that we have largely met the initial intent of this study: to show, in detail, that there are at least a few smaller general hospitals that have psychiatric units that are viable and are perceived to be a valuable resource by and for the community, and within the hospital.

It does not follow, however, that all general hospitals of smaller size should undertake to develop psychiatric units—for a variety of reasons.

Important among these would be the supply of psychiatric beds already available within reasonable distance. Of the ten hospitals that we visited, only two were reasonably proximate to other hospitals having psychiatric units. (Such proximity would not automatically rule out the suitability of starting another, if the existing units were running at or near capacity much of the time; additional psychiatric beds might be a needed and useful addition to the health resources even of a city already having psychiatric units that are heavily utilized.) Apart from these two hospitals, however, the other eight were located at least 25 miles, and up to 60, from any other general hospital having a psychiatric unit. In times when focus on financing is particularly great, it would be unrealistic to argue for establishing a psychiatric unit solely on the grounds that it is preferable to have inpatient treatment available close at hand. Realizing this, we would nonetheless again point out that when a patient whose condition makes hospitalization highly preferable, treatment capability available close enough that relatives and friends—and as frequently happened within some of the units which we visited, employers—can readily visit will for most patients be an advantage. The patient already beset with some condition or disorder requiring that he be isolated from his regular contacts and pursuits will feel less estranged than would be the case were he transported fifty miles from home to a treatment facility. Visits from relatives, particularly, will serve to reinforce the patient's sense that he is being supported and not abandoned, and these visits will give him something to look forward to, so that the passing hours do not seem longer when hospitalized than when in the community.

If the hospital aspires to reidentify itself as a "medical center," as many, including some quite small ones, do these days,

26

the creation within it of a psychiatric unit would certainly be in the interest of the new identity it is striving for.

We have not mentioned earlier the further advantage of having psychiatric physicians available to do consultations for other services of the hospitals. In at least five of the hospitals we visited, the psychiatric physicians were so readily assimilated and integrated into the medical staff that they were frequently called upon to do consultations for physicians of patients in other services of the hospital. Less frequently, but with some regularity, the psychiatrists requested that physicians from the medical and surgical wards do consultations on psychiatric patients. The readiness with which such consultations were sought and given had, in most cases, developed over a period of time, and in some cases as the result of conscious effort; but in some of these hospitals, it seemed clear, psychiatry was viewed not as some interloper or misfit but as fully a part of the medical mission of the facility.

In this same vein, the general hospital administrator and his staff can readily help to reduce the stigma of being treated as a psychiatric patient. Two of our ten hospitals from time to time held open houses and also invited civic groups to use their facilities for meetings, and one of them had held several brief "courses," on such topics as anxiety and depression, for the general public; in the course of such activities and arrangements, visitors had had the opportunity to see the psychiatric unit as an integral, and, to an extent, as "just one other," of the various services which the hospital provided.

*   *   *

The evidently successful incorporation of psychiatric services at Chelsea Community Hospital (p. 103) was notable to those who have seen, at the other extreme from it, considerable "distancing" between "medicine" and "psychiatry." The integration at Chelsea was sufficient to lead to considerable pondering of how it had come about. But the psychiatrist who was chief of service ventured that the psychological distancing of psychiatry in some general hospitals was readily understandable. "It must surely have to do with the unavailability of psychiatrists 'of hospital bent,' together with a prematurely and insufficiently formed idea of 'what psychiatric patients are all about,' and, following from that, an inevitable non-accepting attitude toward them." Psychiatric patients, he felt, are frequently seen as something different from what a community general hospital exists for. "I am sure," he told us, "that not enough people ever really sat down and gave the matter intensive or penetrating thought." He felt that some circumstances at his hospital undoubtedly predisposed an effective identity for psychiatry: the important role that psychiatry played with the patients on the burn unit, with the advanced arthritic patients, and with the relatives of both; the decision to have a single social service department and a single occupational therapy department hospital-wide, flexibly servicing the component units to the extent needed, and adapting their program to make their components suitable for patients in psychiatry; and the practice of having all nurses oriented to a "unihospital" identity. In sum, he felt that at his hospital there was a cultural attitude that the differences within medicine are secondary to the similarities of sensible and adaptable patient care. We were not surprised, when we asked this psychiatrist to state the term which he felt characterized the image of the psychiatry service within the hospital, that he replied, "It's esteemed—now." He also felt strongly that a major factor in its acceptance was the considerable experience that he and his fellow psychiatrist had had in general practice before they did their residencies in psychiatry.

*   *   *

Still to be mentioned is another major impetus to carry out this study. The time may be right for considering establishing a psychiatric unit precisely because, on average, the average census of the community general hospitals has been steadily falling. Without overloading the reader with statistics, suffice it to say that the average census for such hospitals in the early 1960's hovered around the 75 percent mark (and the average census for the psychiatric units of those hospitals was, in those years, fractionally higher, at about 77 percent). By the late 1970's, the average community general hospital census, nationwide, hovered round the 65 percent mark. While this represents an absolute decline of approximately ten percent, when figured from the baseline occupancy rate in the 1960's, the decline amounts to 13 percent. That this drop in average occupancy of beds occurred results from several causes; important among these are the fact that many procedures once invariably done in the hospital are increasingly being done in the doctor's office or in outpatient clinics; and the average length of stay in community general hospitals has declined, for a number of illnesses.

Because a substantial part of the operating expenses of hospitals is largely fixed, falling very little if the census declines, the lower utilization inevitably has forced hospital charges to rise; the percentage of increase in the room-and-board charge of hospitals is among the highest of all commodities in the economy.

In many cases, existing unused wings or floors of general hospitals could be converted at relatively small expense to serve

29

as psychiatric units. Little is needed in the way of costly equipment; if electroconvulsive therapy is to be part of the treatment regimen—and it was not in most of the ten hospitals we visited for this study—the equipment is not expensive. Otherwise, the main special requirement is one of adequate space for the daytime use of patients, most of whom do not require a bed except for nighttime sleeping. Rooms previously used as patient rooms could serve quite well, if interior walls were suitably relocated and if the rooms were appropriately furnished with tables, chairs, and some storage units for reading materials, recreational supplies, and the like; and among the rooms should be one available for group therapeutic meetings with the physician and other staff. At most of the hospitals we visited, the "day room" was also quite satisfactorily set up so that it included, or could be easily converted to, an area for meals. If the unit had no office for physicians and others to use for their paperwork and to see patients individually, a patient room might easily be adapted for such use. Presumably the wing or floor to be converted would have a nursing station, and there seemed to be no imperative specifications for its location except that it have adequate provision for medications, charts, and the like.

The physical facilities of the ten hospitals visited ranged from barely adequate in one case (meaning that the ward was old and cramped and greatly in need of renovation) to exceptionally fine in two hospitals, one of which had had the psychiatric unit "custom designed" when a new physical plant was being planned for the long-established hospital to relocate to; in this attractive unit, all psychiatric patients were housed in single rooms of good size and having connecting baths. The considerable possibility for improvisation, when one does not have the advantage of a custom-designed unit included in the architectural planning, is demonstrated by the fact that one of the ten units we visited was housed in what had been the dormitory of a nursing school that the hospital had formerly run but then shut down, and another in a building attached to the rest of the hospital only by a corridor and built to serve as a nursing home, which failed financially when newer nursing homes were constructed in its immediate vicinity.

That there have been in recent years, in some parts of the country, extreme strictures upon what hospitals may do, extending even in some places to the modification of existing facilities without significant expenditure, the authors are well aware. The health service agencies have varied, as any large group of agencies is apt to do, from extremely powerful in some places to having relatively little effect in other parts of the country. The authority of these agencies appears to be in decline; but we began this study at a time when we fully understood that their power was so great in some locales that they could have blocked the establishment of psychiatric units even by converting unused space and even when existing psychiatric resources in community hospitals were running a high census most of the time and were entirely filled some of the time; but we knew that there were areas where these agencies would have been less rigid.

Any small hospital considering whether it would be suitable to establish a psychiatric unit would obviously want to feel assured that, beyond the percent of occupancy that might be anticipated, the clientele would have the means to pay for services rendered. As this is written, in late 1982, it is undoubtedly the most problematic factor. Some of the ten programs we visited were receiving some public reimbursement, usually for specific services rendered—and in one state at a rate considerably lower than the hospital's expenditures, and in another state under an authorization which the legislature in some years did not appropriate money to cover. In addition to cuts already effected in both federal and state health support programs, there is pervasive talk that further cuts will be made, soon and again later. Beyond this, the "benefit package" of some private health insurance plans has been cut and there is pervasive talk of further cuts to come. Presumably any hospital's administrator and board would take cognizance of these developments and would ponder further developments that are under discussion. The time available during our visits to these hospitals did not allow any detailed exploration of the sources of payments. It may be sufficient to say that the majority of all services being rendered was being paid by third parties, public or private, and it seems unlikely that more than a small percentage of the population would be able to pay from their personal resources for more than a brief inpatient stay in any service of a general hospital.

Finally, an effective psychiatric unit must have a competent, well-integrated, and well-trained staff. We see this as perhaps the smallest of the problems involved in initiating a psychiatric unit in a general hospital. None of these ten visited in this study—even the most remote and the sparest of them—had experienced any significant difficulty in recruiting staff of evidently good quality, well informed about the field, personable, efficient, and appropriately invested in their work.

PART II

Psychiatric Services in
Seven Smaller General Hospitals

Mercy Medical Center
Roseburg, Oregon

JUST OVER A CENTURY ago, "seven young Sisters of Mercy brought their mission across the Mississippi and into the West," says Mercy Medical Center's beautiful and tasteful brochure, enlivened with many large color photographs.

Roseburg, Oregon, where Mercy Medical Center is located, had in 1979 about 20,000 residents. It is a little more than an hour's drive south from Eugene (population about 100,000) and a little more than a three-hour drive from Portland (population about 350,000). Roseburg is more or less the same size as other towns in the southern part of the state. "Settled" about 130 years ago, Roseburg serves the lumber industry, whose mills and plywood plants process the trees cut from extensive stands of virgin timber. There are also some vineyards and vineries in the vicinity. A national forest and a state park in the proximity offer plentiful opportunity for fishing, camping, and hiking. Roseburg is the seat of and market center for Douglas County (population about 88,000). It is a prosperous-looking town, clean and pleasant, set within rolling hills, and close by to low mountains. If it is not trendy or chic, nor aspiring to be, it has the aura of a place where life is orderly and people are mindful of the needs and rights of others, and where the clean air makes for easy breathing. Only an hour away, at Eugene's airport, getaways are daily available via non-stop flights to Los Angeles, San Francisco, and Seattle, plus through flights to Atlanta, Denver, Phoenix, Portland, and Tucson.

One local resident told us, "Roseburg is a good place to bring up kids." It is conservative, and a psychiatrist told us that "what is expected of people is a little more than in the average community." The population was increasing, and there was a sense of "growing pains." A psychologist on Mercy's psychiatric unit told us that the county has "a contingent of young people without families, without jobs, without an established place to live. Some of them tend to be loners, estranged from their families, and some consume much alcohol and various other drugs." Some of these grew up in Roseburg, and others relocated to it. Said the hospital's social service director, "We are not without some really mixed up younger people, who find themselves in situations beyond their control."

As modern, attractive, and well equipped as is Mercy Medical Center itself, Roseburg, for a town of its size and locus, has had an impressive extent of other medical facilities. The only other general hospital for the general public is Douglas Community Hospital, with 135 beds—some 24 more than at Mercy. Its average occupancy had been notably low—only a little over fifty percent—and it had no psychiatric service and is notable to this report mainly because it was in process of assuming the function of detoxifying alcoholics, something that Mercy had previously done but had arranged to be relieved of doing, in part because of the ample availability of beds at Douglas and also because the state's reimbursement rate for alcohol detoxification was considerably less than what Mercy had found it necessary to spend. A third general hospital in Roseburg is operated by the Veterans Administration. It was at one time a neuropsychiatric hospital but it had been reclassified by the Veterans Administration as a "long-stay general hospital," with more beds than Mercy and Douglas combined and an average occupancy of 85 percent. Other than in Roseburg, hospitals in Douglas County are very small. There are general hospitals of moderate size in adjacent counties, but the only one with a psychiatric unit is some sixty miles from Roseburg and consequently even less accessible to most Douglas County residents than the general hospital psychiatry service in Eugene.

In 1977, Mercy Medical Center's new 111-bed plant was finished, at a new site at the edge of Roseburg, in the main direction in which the city was extending. It fully deserved to call itself "medical center," having a highly advanced coronary unit, a maternity program that begins with expectant couples and involves the whole family through and beyond delivery, and advanced ambulance service working in concert with a 24-hour emergency room, and such technology as echocardiography, the gamma camera of nuclear medicine, and home health care delivered by a team of nurses who go to patients' homes to change dressings, give medications, and do "health teaching" to patients and families. The hospital had two full-time physical therapists. Except in pediatrics, there were no traditional nursing stations but rather "pod nursing," with supplies and medicines packaged and delivered by cart to each service. Food services, the supply system, and all else were of a quality that beggers the word "modern." The building itself, of clean angular lines and surrounded by sloping lawns, was as unusually attractive as the brochure that presents it. On the ground floor was the psychiatric service, with its ten private rooms; the hospital's brochure does not mention it, or the word psychiatry, or the term mental health. Nonetheless, psychiatric beds were by no means an afterthought; they were included in the plans from the outset.

The mental health unit, as the psychiatry service was called, had been fully described in a separate brochure, front and back of a legal-sized sheet, illustrated with several photographs. It gave a good general description of the unit (which is an open unit), and fairly full information about treatments, staffing, admission policy, handling of emergencies, and dispositions available for patients being discharged. It states—correctly, we felt—that the unit, comprising a self-contained wing, is "a comfortable, attractive, and therapeutic environment for the psychiatric care and treatment of both inpatients and outpatients." This unit, it continues, offers (only) private rooms, with private toilet facilities and telephones, features a restful view of the landscape, and has color television. "Special areas in the unit accommodate planned group meetings and individual therapy. A sunny recreation room and the outdoors facilitate socialization and a variety of recreational pursuits, such as Ping Pong, volleyball, outdoor gatherings, and walks." That one group room is converted, efficiently and with dispatch, to a dining room three times per day. It might be considered "skimpy" as gathering space were it not for the facts that patients have abundant-sized private rooms, the average stay is short (seven days), and there are frequent out-of-hospital activities. The unit also has two offices for physician-patient interviews. In the "educational room" used by the entire hospital, movies are shown for psychiatric patients and others.

Two of the ten rooms had security features sufficient for significantly agitated and potentially dangerous patients. We were told that, over a considerable period of time, these had been used mainly for alcoholism patients needing to be withdrawn under supervision, but such patients were increasingly being handled by Douglas Community Hospital.

The psychiatry brochure lists as grounds for admission: *a*) severe behavior disorders which endanger the life of the patient or others; *b*) severe mental illness and disorganized behavior; *c*) psychosomatic symptoms requiring intensive psychiatric treatment; *d*) inability to deal with the realities and requirements of home and/or work while undergoing outpatient therapy.

* * *

The Staff. Dr. Saeed Aflatooni is a psychiatrist who arranged, seemingly to his own satisfaction and to the advantage of the hospital, to be chief of service. Trained in psychiatry in his native Iran, he repeated his training at Nebraska Psychiatric Institute. He soon thereafter sought an opportunity simultaneously to develop an office practice and to develop a broad-range general hospital psychiatric unit in an area with a good climate. Having learned about the opening at Mercy, he relocated to Roseburg in mid-1978. For heading the inpatient service he received no salary.

Since the state of Oregon by statute serves as payer of last resort for a maximum of 12 days of local psychiatric hospitalization, there was no great financial risk. The county mental health department was the agent recipient of the funds, which would not cover treatment of physical illness, nor of persons in process of commitment proceedings, nor electroshock treatment (which was not used at Mercy).

Dr. Aflatooni had developed what seemed to be a sensible team approach. He met with the team, most days of the week, in the morning, again just after lunch, and then again for evening rounds. Since his outpatient practice was done from an attractive office in a medical office building a block away, he was conveniently close. He worked with and got assistance from and gave assistance to a psychiatrist recently recruited by the county mental health program and also an older psychiatrist, who, as part of "phasing down," had relocated to Roseburg several years earlier to work part time. This man came when only a family clinic had a psychiatrist. In those days management-problem patients, according to size of problem, were held either in jail or in a makeshift room in the county nursing home, awaiting transfer to the state hospital 130 miles away, unless patient or family could pay for and preferred transfer to a voluntary hospital fifty miles away in Eugene. To the state hospital went "the insane," whereas manageable, reasonably cooperative cases were housed in Mercy's regular medical wards. While it was still at its earlier facility, Mercy Hospital designated two medical rooms for psychiatric patients and had experienced not a few problems. The area's sole psychiatrist departed and the county health officer filled in, with some help from the recently arrived "phasing down" psychiatrist. By the time of our visit, the county clinic had acquired a full-time psychiatrist, and also a child psychiatrist had relocated to Roseburg to set up an office practice.

*   *   *

The stigma of mental illness seemed notably less in Roseburg than in most places we have been. Since the Veterans Administration general hospital had once been entirely psychiatric, the townspeople were accustomed to seeing "these neuropsychiatric people" around town. But at Mercy's previous facility, its two-bed allocation for psychiatry was referred to as "the funny place." At the new facility, we were told, psychiatry had become "one part of the hospital, in the same way that obstetrics is one part."

The admission policy allowed any physician on the hospital staff to admit to psychiatry, and some did, freely using Dr. Aflatooni as consultant; while others referred the patient to him.

The psychiatric unit had coverage by registered nurses at all times, with four of them thus having to divvy up the week to an average of 42 hours on duty. The head nurse had a master's degree in psychiatric nursing. There were one full-time and one part-time licensed practical nurses and seven assistants or "techs." Until recently before our visit, a full-time occupational therapist had divided her time between psychiatry and the adjacent physical therapy section, and, since she had resigned, a replacement was being sought. Dr. Aflatooni's wife, with an Iranian degree in psychology and an American degree in community service counseling, worked half time, among other things leading the twice-weekly group therapy. Another employee, also with a degree in community counseling, was head of hospital–wide social service but spent much of her time with psychiatric patients.

The head nurse, after having worked for a dozen years on surgical and neurosurgical services elsewhere, had "got enthused about" more training, and in San Francisco had earned a B.A. in behavioral sciences and an M.A. in rehabilitation counseling. She had had considerable experience in psychiatric, detoxification, and terminal units before coming to Roseburg, arriving there not very long before our visit. It was her conscious choice to turn her back on super-urbia and seek out an appealing setting in the Northwest. In the short time she had been at Mercy, she had found the experience simultaneously exhausting, satisfying, and fulfilling. "I am doing education, and one-to-one intensive counseling, and group therapy, and simultaneously, in every sense, being a nurse," she told us. "Yes, it is certainly fulfilling."

Inservice training. There had been some inservice training and more was planned. Dr. Aflatooni had taught, within the hospital, a course on clinical psychiatry, rich in content, consisting of weekly sessions for 16 weeks. The hospital gave the staff on duty release time to attend, and it also compensated those who came in for the sessions during off-duty hours.

As for intra-hospital relationships, an attending general practitioner told us that he thought patients with emotional or mental illness had come to fare much better. "Although I have no particular knowledge in counseling, I used to spend much time doing counseling—for instance, a husband and wife in a troubled marriage—but I find that nowadays people are more willing to accept a referral to a psychiatrist, particularly when one is available here in town and not at a distance of fifty miles. In my own practice women are more willing, sometimes eager, to be referred, the men definitely more resistant. Anyway, this psychiatric service has certainly taken a load off my shoulders. The psychiatrists seem able to establish rapport readily. I occasionally ask Dr. Aflatooni to consult on one of my hospitalized patients, and my colleagues sometimes do, too. And it works in both directions. When Dr. Aflatooni finds that a patient he's treating has medical problems, he calls the primary physician and asks him to do a consultation in the psychiatry unit." He added that he felt that most of the medical staff were delighted that the psychiatric unit was part of the hospital. Nurses and technicians on the medical services, he added, "used to be afraid of psychiatric patients, but most of them have become interested and enthusiastic."

*   *   *

The patients. All patients at Mercy Hospital were assured of rights consistent with those promulgated by the National Conference of Catholic Bishops. They include the right to obtain from the physician "complete current information concerning diagnosis, treatment, and prognosis, in terms the patient can be reasonably expected to understand," or, if a patient's condition makes this inadvisable, the information is furnished in his behalf to a relative or some other appropriate person. The patient may refuse treatment "to the extent permitted by law" and must be informed of the medical consequences thereof. He is entitled to "every consideration" of his privacy. Case discussion, consultation, examination, and treatment "are confidential and will be conducted discreetly." All communications and records are treated as confidential.

Psychiatric patients had a heavier—we felt appropriately heavier—program than in some longer established and better-known units. Patients rose at 6:00 for usual personal hygiene and grooming, then met for breakfast at 7:30, then had a half-hour exercise period. This was followed three days per week by a "gestalt group" led by Dr. Aflatooni, then followed by his rounds on patients and others, followed by an hour of arts and crafts. On the two intermediate days, he saw patients individually. This was followed on one day by an hour's "communication group" and on the other day by an hour's music therapy, each of which was followed by a half-hour activity out-of-doors. At eleven o'clock three mornings per week was a patient education group using a "board talk" devised by the head nurse and the other two mornings by a remotivation group led by Ms. Aflatooni. After a brief lunch, there was a group meeting, Monday through Friday, called "Growth and Change," followed by another half hour out of doors, followed by two hours of rest time, followed by an hour of group recreation. Dinner was then served, at 5:00, and followed by visiting hours, up to 8:00 o'clock. At that hour, three days per week, there was a group session, and on two other days a "relaxation group." Nine o'clock was bedtime. This schedule, and much more in the way of information useful to patients, was handily set forth in a folder provided to each patient. It included details of privilege levels, which range from essentially none at level one up to passes and home visits at level three. To achieve level three, the patient must keep himself and his room clean and neat, attend scheduled events and get to them on time, help get things ready for events and clean up afterward, take prescribed medications, and refrain from physical or verbal abuse and from monopolizing the telephone.

*   *   *

Of 470 patients discharged during the first year of operation, the final diagnoses were: schizophrenia, 30 percent; alcoholism, 17 percent, and mental disorder associated with alcohol, another 11 percent; neuroses, 14 percent; personality disorders, six percent; major affective disorders, five percent; and transient situational disorders, three percent. There were two percent each of mental disorder with drugs, chronic brain syndrome, drug abuse, and behavior disorder of childhood. Thirteen persons were scattered among eight other diagnoses. Those patients having been previously hospitalized for the same diagnosis represented 45 percent of personality disorders, forty percent of schizophrenics, forty percent of alcoholics, 36 percent of major affective disorders, 33 percent of neuroses, and 27 percent of those with mental disorder associated with alcohol.

The average stay during that first year was only six days; it was longer than ten days only for the diagnoses of adjustment reaction (11 days, three persons) and psychosis specific to childhood (19 days, two persons). For the first four months of 1979, neuroses had risen to the modal diagnosis and schizophrenia had fallen to second place, the average stay had risen by less than half a day, and only two categories of diagnosis representing seven patients averaged a stay longer than ten days; of course, we are reporting relatively small numbers of cases over a short time period.

When we visited, there were patients who had recently been through horrendous experiences. One operator of heavy machinery had had a serious accident and had become phobic about the machinery essential to his work. What benefit might he get? "He is getting some time out, which he needs, both because of the accident and also because of persistent family friction, and he is getting appropriate medication for his severe insomnia. He is in the midst of sympathetic and supportive people, and nobody is ridiculing him." Another patient was very nearly dysfunctional because of grief over her husband's accidental death; she had progressed through denial and anger, but was then contemplating suicide. She was getting support, empathy, and light medication. The staff, some with experience in a variety of kinds of communities and cities, did not feel that patients were admitted casually and needlessly.

If a patient were employed, and if he consented, Ms. Aflatooni got in touch with his supervisor, and "usually they keep their jobs." A lot of them, she added, "don't have jobs to start with."

* * *

Emergencies. Persons thought likely to be dangerous to themselves or others, or unable to care for themselves, as an evident result of mental illness, were placed under "police officer hold," presented for immediate physician examination, and, if the doctor determined the person to be "in need of immediate psychiatric care," taken to Mercy Hospital's emergency room; it was stipulated that the "peace officer will remain with the person . . . until he is safely in bed in the security unit."

Mercy's emergency room was staffed by full-time emergency room physicians. One of them expressed his mixed feelings about psychiatric patients brought there. "One feeling," he said, "is fairly selfish. Specifically, the patients, most of them brought by the police, take up more time and are often extremely disruptive in an emergency department that is frequently full. The positive side, despite what I've just said, is to see such patients, who had been brought here disturbed many times, admitted to psychiatry and later coming back mainly with physical problems, and seeming to be doing well in psychiatric respects. Psychiatry is still new, but we are starting already to get some real benefits from it." The acting-up (or acting-out) patients he had described, he said, "are treated well by the police, with respect and kindness. The presence of the uniform makes a big difference and keeps many of them in line until they can be medicated." He said that quite a few were people "being combative with cars out on the freeway, or they've shot up their neighbor's property, and many are strung out—probably well over half, if you add up drugs and alcohol plus a combination of the two." Such persons averaged from two to three a week. The most difficult were those who seemed reasonably controlled until the police left, "when all hell breaks loose—to the point that the patient is so dangerously uncontrollable it's practically impossible to medicate him." Sometimes hospital staff telephoned the police to ask that they reappear, and occasionally a patient was taken to the holding room at the jail. The emergency room physicians could use whatever medication was necessary, and mechanical restraint as well. All patients must be either discharged from the emergency room or admitted to the hospital; there was no provision or space for an overnight or other extended hold for observation.

* * *

Financing. The county paid for an initial five days of involuntary treatment unless it was proposed to the patient, and he agreed, that he be converted to voluntary status, at which point the county would no longer pay. County payment could be extended with approval for as many as seven days additional to the initial five. The head nurse in psychiatry met regularly with county health department personnel to review financial status and exchange pertinent information about recently admitted patients.

* * *

Community education. Dr. Aflatooni, hoping to do well for the unit while ministering to the community, had made several presentations for the general public—on depression, stress, and parenting. The local newspaper and radio station announced the events. Dr. Aflatooni and a person charged with public education on behalf of the entire hospital had appeared on local television for a 15-minute interview about a forthcoming depression presentation, done in a single evening. The first time offered, 140 people came, more than could be seated in the conference room. For the second, 101 came.

Already planned were future presentations on stress and on relaxation, and also the hospital had been approached by the school system with the request to set up a youth group "for some of the troubled teenagers they are counseling."

* * *

Future aspirations. The absolutely good and relatively great acceptance of this service suggested it had good, perhaps great expectations. It was widely and appropriately valued; despite those who, to avoid stigma, preferred to go away for treatment, the unit was likely to do a good volume—although, as with most psychiatric units, there was great variability in the census. From all we could learn, other physicians were remarkably accepting of, or, at minimum, of benign attitude towards, psychiatry. Plans were well underway for a day care center, intended to be used largely by ex-patients and to some extent by present patients and outpatients; it would be located conveniently, since the physical therapy department neighboring psychiatry was slated to be relocated and its vacated space would serve as the day care quarters. Referrals to the state hospital from this county had dropped from well over a hundred per year in the mid-1970's to 26 persons the year before we visited—a decrease of about 80 percent.

In summary. We felt this unit to be as impressive as it was small. It was staffed with people who had good formal training or adequate and appropriate on-the-job training. It accepted a broad range of problems and persons. It had for patients a program full enough and varied enough to be a credit to any such unit, and one that some larger prestigious, big-city hospitals would do well to contemplate. Although disturbed patients sometimes made trouble in the emergency room, that was where they were brought rather than being isolated ("stigmatized") by way of a separate service. The length of inpatient stay was very short, yet few patients were transferred to other inpatient facilities. The day program being planned would provide for some patients an important form of after-care. Every town and county of this physical size and population would be fortunate to have such a service.

Flagler Hospital
St. Augustine, Florida

S T. AUGUSTINE is a small town—about 15,000 inhabitants in
1981—which has much in common with other somewhat
isolated small towns, even though its early development, some
decades ago, was spurred by tourism. In the heyday of passenger trains, St. Augustine was for a time the end of the East
Coast line, and there railroad magnate Henry Flagler built two
ornate and elaborate hotels and several neighboring buildings in
neospanish style, near the vast fort which Spanish colonizers
had built a great deal earlier. While today's St. Augustine is
visited, usually briefly, by many tourists en route to newer and
livelier resorts, mainly it is home to retirees, and its businesses
are small ones to meet their needs. The grounds of the larger of
the once bustling hotels are now those of a small college. A
bridge nearby spans the bay, to the upper end of a peninsula
surrounded by beaches and dotted with a few resort motels of
recent advent, patronized mostly by summer vacationers.

Around the beginning of this century, Flagler Hospital was
established at the southern end of the town of St. Augustine,
and it functioned for seventy years as the only general hospital
in its county. Specialized procedures which it did not perform

required an hour's journey north to Jacksonville. In a three-county area there were no psychiatric or mental health services of any kind, and persons in need of them either went north to Jacksonville, south to Daytona Beach, west to private services in Gainesville (where the University of Florida and its medical school are located), or, if they lacked means, were held in jail awaiting transport to the nearest state hospital, about fifty miles away.

In 1972 Florida's legislature passed an act providing a degree of fiscal support for treating alcoholics, and another mandating local treatment for mental patients and providing payment at a modest rate for as much as 15 days of inpatient treatment for those having no other source of funds. In St. Augustine, Flagler Hospital was showing its age, and talk was growing of the interest of a group of doctors in building not far away a new general hospital which they would own. Flagler's generally low census and the talk of impending competition were factors in its decision to designate a few of its beds as a psychiatric unit.

For two years the newly established unit operated with general physicians admitting and attending psychiatric patients, in collaboration with a medically retired ex-Navy psychiatrist who served as chief of service and consultant. This psychiatrist remained at Flagler until 1975. In the meantime, in 1973, G. R. Baringer, who had been a member of the staff of a large and active university hospital, relocated to St. Augustine, because he felt he would enjoy "a less energy- and resource-draining locale, particularly with ready access to ocean, shore, and nature." When the retired Navy captain relinquished his affiliation with Flagler, a friend of Baringer's came to St. Augustine to head up the Flagler unit, among other things, and persuaded Baringer to share the responsibility with him. In 1977 this latest arrived psychiatrist moved to Gainesville to become director of inpatient services at the University of Florida's Department of Psychiatry. Dr. Baringer thereafter ran the Flagler unit alone, until, some months later, he convinced another psychiatrist to join forces. She and Dr. Baringer shared duties, income, and office practice until mid-1979.

This latest-to-arrive psychiatrist handled the inpatient unit medically on her own for some months, and then departed. Dr. Baringer, the sole psychiatrist on the St. Augustine scene throughout these years, attributed the succession of other psychiatrists to "chronic economic discontent," since the provisions of the state's mandated treatment act had not been adjusted financially since inception and the reimbursement for physicians was very small. He urged the hospital, as a means of dealing with the frequently re-emerging problem, to establish a salaried, almost half-time, position for chief of service, although he declined to accept it—on the grounds that the amount of paper work, the restrictions, and the formalities had proliferated beyond the bent of a psychiatrist who was "not very political"; and in any case, he had wanted all along to concentrate his time on private outpatient work, he being the only such practitioner within a fifty-mile radius of St. Augustine.

But no other psychiatrist being attracted by the job, Baringer felt a responsibility to fill in until one could be recruited, and so he was doing at the point that we visited the hospital, in 1979.

Intercurrently an expansion of mental health services for the county, and two adjacent counties, had become possible by means of an NIMH community mental health center grant awarded to the three-county area. At the time of our visit, "Tri-County," as the catchment area was known, was utilizing Flagler Hospital for psychiatric inpatient care and was operating its own alcohol detoxification center, a halfway house, a program for day patients, and three small outpatient clinics—one in each county.

* * *

During the several prior years, any physician on Flagler's staff could, by hospital policy and practice, admit patients to psychiatry. Those physicians who rotated on hospital-wide emergency back-up coverage occasionally were presented with an emergency psychiatric patient, in some cases brought by the police, whom they felt there was reason to admit to psychiatry—and then, as hospital policy prescribed, to follow.

The events thus had unfolded as improbably as events usually do. Baringer was attracted to the small-town life style and setting of St. Augustine, where he wished to practice psychiatry privately but not to head up a general hospital inpatient unit. He nonetheless agreed to do so for a time, when local needs so pointed. But in no great time, he was devoting more of his hours to an inpatient service and less to an office practice than he had ever intended. Eventually a "successor" as head of the hospital inpatient service came, then went, and so did another. All this while any physician on the Flagler attending staff could by policy admit psychiatric patients, and to some extent did, not always with complete comfort or confidence. (When the new physician-owned general hospital opened, some of Flagler's attending physicians relocated to it exclusively, but most physicians chose to be on the attending staff of both hospitals.)

* * *

When we visited Flagler, we entered an old but considerably renovated hospital, with bright and attractive lounges, offices, and patient rooms, divided among medical and surgical, pediatric, obstetrical, and intensive care services. Then we arrived at the time-worn, dreary, and cramped psychiatric unit, accommodating up to nine patients in triple rooms, and if needed, an additional two or three through improvising the arrangements. There was a cramped nursing station, a cheerless "lounge" that doubled as dining room, and, at a slight remove, another room in process of becoming an activities area. The ward was unlocked except when there was an evidently elope-prone involuntary or "risky" patient. While voluntary patients could sign out against medical advice, with no waiting period, it was hoped each such would make known his intention to leave and agree to sign the "AMA" form. Passes to go alone to the snack shop or to walk on the grounds were generously granted. Visiting hours were generous on weekends and skimpy on weekdays. Psychiatry ran a significantly higher rate of occupancy than the rest of the hospital and did better financially, yet had physical facilities that were no better than acceptable and too small. This spartan unit was scheduled for eventual renovation; apparently this was to be the last to be upgraded because of the need to make the other services more comparable to those of the new general hospital—which would not accept psychiatric admissions.

*   *   *

The entry point. The Tri-County clinics were the designated standard point of psychiatric entry—except that about a quarter of psychiatric patients came or were brought by relatives or police to Flagler's emergency room. Should staff of one of the Tri-County clinics decide inpatient treatment was indicated, the patient was given a referral slip and sent or, if necessary, transported to Flagler. The emergency room physician could decline to admit if he felt that inpatient care was not needed, but that rarely happened. Grounds for admission were numerous and broad. Perhaps deserving of notice were "inadequate social support" and "shallowness or lability of affect." If the police brought the patient, they might "be required" to accompany him to the inpatient service "and asked to remain as long as necessary." Patients could be admitted, for not more than 48 hours, against their wishes. Those unwilling to sign themselves in were given notice of right of *habeas corpus,* and the court of competence had to be notified within a stipulated 48 hours "not counting weekends." Thus, it might not be unfair to say that the written procedure, here as in most other services, for detaining (protecting) a patient "with due legal process" was more accurately a "procedure for detaining protesting patients for evaluation or observation." Of the attending physicians, there were some five who served to cover out-of-hours psychiatric cases, only one of whom chose to write orders, the others deferring to Baringer for a "consultation," whereby it was he who wrote orders.

*   *   *

The patient mix was varied. Of 25 patients consecutively admitted shortly before our visit, two had Medicare coverage, one had Blue Cross insurance, and the remaining 22 would be cared for under state support. Of the 25, thirteen had a schizophrenia diagnosis; seven were diagnosed as depressed; and there were one each diagnosed as manic-depressive, alcoholic with risk of DT's, adolescent adjustment reaction, situational reaction, and "psychotic episode." Twelve of the 25 had been previously hospitalized on psychiatric bases one or more times.

More than half had been "after-hours" (i.e. night or weekend) admissions.

Four were transferred to the state hospital.

It seemed clear that most patients were poor, but not covered by Medicaid as rendered in Florida.

A staff member invariably interviewed the patient and family jointly at the time of or shortly after admission. A large number, we were told, were "personality-characterologic" disordered, who came in greatly stressed, sometimes aggressive, sometimes hysterical, sometimes having gestured suicide. The majority were women, most of them married, many unhappily. Baringer told us he supposed such events as wrist–slashing "had become much more visible as facilities were developed to deal with them," and such behavior was now identified as "sick" rather than "mean" or "bad." There were occasional admissions—as we were similarly to hear at most hospitals near an interstate high- way—of patients known as "interstate screamers," generalized as younger people "who figure some sunshine will fix them up, but they begin to go sour around New Jersey and freak out near the Florida line and run naked down the median strip." Some of these were clearly drug freak-outs.

But it was rarely necessary to seclude any patient because he was unmanageable or presumably suicidal; when this was done, it was required that a staff member check on the patient each 15 minutes. In general, the staff seemed adept at "mellowing down" a variety of agitated, poorly controlled patients. "Usu- ally," one nurse told us, "we've been able on first contact to convey to the patient what we're like, what we have in mind for him, and what we expect of him." Most patients were co- operative, although most—at least when we visited—looked fairly disorganized. That might be because Baringer preferred to medicate conservatively.

"It scares me when I think how many of the drugs being prescribed may have long-term adverse effects we don't yet know about,'' Baringer told us; he added that ''maybe it's a natural phenomenon for people to get out of emotional harness from time to time.'' He cited one of the studies finding that the incidence of treating is related to the nearness of treatment facilities. He wondered whether ''we are identifying more cases or simply providing an avenue of expression not previously available.'' He observed that the staff ''has a high tolerance for disturbed behavior, but should we get overloaded at one time, I try to do some shifting around. I'd hate to see that natural tolerance destroyed—or to see the staff resort to shielding themselves behind the nurses station.'' We observed that he was in a sense an orchestrator. He agreed. And one who looked forward to the arrival of still another full-time inpatient psychiatrist so that he could relinquish these duties. As for the practicality of medically staffing a psychiatric unit with general practice or family practice physicians and only consultation, albeit generous, from a psychiatrist, ''I think it's possible,'' he said, ''but it takes a great deal of faith and attention on everybody's part and quite a lot of motivation.''

One nurse told us that St. Augustine appeared to have more tolerance for disordered behavior than other areas, both small-town and city, where she had worked—but less than it had previously, in part because retirees were moving down from other kinds of places. Even so, St. Augustine's residents were still mainly a mix of retired older conservatives and young conservatives who grew up there. People seemed generally ''accepting'' of their circumstances and many would perhaps be considered elsewhere to have a touch of chronic depression.

The inpatient staff. This small unit seemed adequately staffed. Of the two RN's, one was trained in psychiatry; each had on her shift an LPN and one or two aides. At night, there was an

LPN, an aide, and an orderly. The total ratio, at full occupancy, was 1.5 staff per patient.

*　　*　　*

In-hospital relationships. The attending physicians who admitted and followed psychiatric patients did so because it was expected more than because they found it satisfying.

Occasionally, Baringer was asked to do a consultation on a patient in a medical ward, and occasionally a significantly distressed medical ward patient was transferred to psychiatry, "treated understandingly," and quickly returned. Nurses on other services, once decidedly aloof "because they feared what they didn't understand," were less so, but still were not assigned to fill in for or to augment psychiatric staff. There was still the occasional "incident"—a wandering psychiatric patient who became boisterous in the hospital lounge, for example—that kept some sense of "differentness" alive.

For the most part, psychiatric nursing staff at Flagler had already been working elsewhere in the hospital and had "self-selected" themselves into psychiatry. The morale was good. "Even the maid proves helpful through conversing with patients." Baringer described the unit "as a milieu therapy of a kind," wherein all employees, most patients, and most relatives in combination provided what might be called multiple family therapy, for all but heavily medicated or highly agitated patients.

But he was emphatically concerned that some proportion of staff must be thoroughly trained. "Training is critical; one should 'get in deep' by working deeply for a time with a few patients, and internalize that experience, because it enables one to operate more adequately in a short-term service." He thought some experience in an outpatient setting was also important. "This is how one acquires the attitude that 'I'm responsible *to'*—not *for*—this person." Conservative medication, consistent observation, a "milieu approach," the involvement of relatives, and some outdoor activities were the substance of the program. (A Flagler College student was there on placement, as one frequently was, serving mainly as an activities aide, encouraging patients to participate in games or "classes.") The "psychotherapy" was perceived as "counseling," as dealing with present manifest problems, with little delving, as one put it, that would concentrate on making the patients more insightful about what they do.

ECT was unavailable at Flagler, rarely indicated for its patients in Baringer's opinion, and a course of it administered at a distant facility when necessary—usually two or three times a year. For Flagler's psychiatric patients, social service assistance was provided, to some extent, by the staff of the Tri-County mental health unit. (Flagler Hospital had no social worker at all.)

*　　*　　*

The conscientious director of the Tri-County program, a psychologist, came to the Flagler inpatient unit every morning. Since the majority of patients entered via the Tri-County units, they went back there for post-hospital outpatient appointments as needed or to its day program. Many inpatients were also invited upon discharge to return to the inpatient unit on any of three mornings each week. "Quite a few of them do for a while; it's very helpful for present patients to have former patients drop in and talk about how they're doing," one of the nurses told us. Tri-County could arrange for those patients unable to return home to enter its halfway house. Frail elderly persons were usually placed in nursing homes.

Inpatient results. This small unit had been open a little more than five years, as of the time we visited. The population of the three-county area had *increased* during that time by about fifty percent, yet state hospital patient days from these counties had been *reduced* by fifty percent—at least in part because of Flagler's inpatient unit.

Alcoholism. As we heard everywhere we went, there was a great deal of heavy drinking. When it was determined that a patient's problem was "mere" alcoholism—that is, that there seemed to be no germane underlying cause—he was not admitted to the psychiatry unit. Tri-County's Twin Oaks facility was used as a sober-up locus unless there appeared to be a likelihood that delirium tremens would ensue. Detoxification was also done at a small one-time motel which some former alcoholics had acquired. The sheriff, we were told, actively encouraged such facilities because there were potential major legal complications from putting drunk people in jail.

The Mental Health Association. This small county had a mental health association operated entirely by volunteers, who contributed 2,800 hours in the year prior to our visit. It provided day-time telephone consultation, in most cases referring the caller to some part of the Tri-County service. One volunteer solicited good used clothing for the alcoholics dried out at Twin Oaks. The group made Christmas gifts for patients at Flagler, Twin Oaks, and the state hospital, and gave parties twice each year for state hospital patients.

Conclusions. This psychiatric unit, in terms of physical facilities and condition the plainest and sparest we saw in our visits, gave us a good feeling. While we wished it were not physically so impoverished, the attitude and the competence of the staff we felt were impressively good. The staff were sometimes discouraged by the considerable number of readmissions, yet it was not clear that a longer inpatient stay or any of various other possible changes would assure greater or more enduring improvement. Much good was being accomplished with meager resources. Despite the apparent ease with which hospital and Tri-County worked together, the medical identity of the inpatient service seemed clear—evidenced, perhaps most of all, by the fact that nursing staff wore nursing uniforms, so that, as one person remarked, "In this unit, you can readily tell the patients from the staff." Dr. Baringer, interim director because he felt it was his responsibility, seemed clearly to be an intelligent and well-trained man, highly likeable—with an inquiring mind intrigued by moon phases and nutrition. St. Augustine seemed fortunate to have the Flagler psychiatric unit, and the unit fortunate to have Dr. Baringer. If it was a small story, it was a success story.

Subsequently

Dr. Donal Conley had accepted the job of director of inpatient services and had arranged independent status for the nursing service. Personnel otherwise had changed very little. The unit had been not only renovated but expanded to twice its prior bed capacity.

Tulare View Inpatient Service
of
Kings-Tulare Community Mental Health Center
Tulare, California

IN CALIFORNIA, locally based and delivered mental health services are more the product of state legislation than of impetus from the later federal community mental health centers
program. While in some localities services were created, augmented, and in some particulars supported when federal staffing grants became available, the momentum for local programs
was already well begun—starting in the late 1950's, when the
California legislature enacted legislation (the Short-Doyle Act)
whereby state funds would finance one-half of county expenditures for county-operated mental health services. But the counties were not obliged to participate, and a considerable number
did not. Later, when the state increased its share of the cost to
75 percent, some of the county-based programs expanded, and
additional counties began to participate. In time, the state share
went to ninety percent. A main purpose was to provide a range
of treatments near to home, obviating the need to hospitalize the
patient in a state facility which in many cases was some fifty or
hundred miles away from where he lived. A main result, it was
supposed by many, would be a reduction in state hospital pop-

ulation such as to make it possible to reduce both the number and the role of state hospitals.*

Interested and active in the evolution of state support to county mental health services was the Kings View Corporation. It had developed out of a small private psychiatric hospital, Kings View, created as adjunctive to the Mennonite Church. The interest was longstanding. During World War II, some 1,300 Mennonite "conscientious objectors" were assigned for their "alternate service" to various understaffed state mental hospitals, where they were appalled by the crowding, the attitudes, and much more. They urged, following the War, that the Mennonite Church take some action—which it did, by approving the creation of a small private hospital in Western Maryland, then a second, known as Kings View, in the village of Reedley, in Fresno County, California, and, later, another one in California and others in Kansas, in Indiana, and in Canada, in the province of Manitoba.

Kings View Hospital, with 29 beds, opened in 1951, with considerable local support. By the late 1970's, with 55 beds, this well-regarded private psychiatric hospital stayed full and had a waiting list. It provides intermediate length "reconstructive" inpatient psychiatric care. The patients come, in many cases, from other states. This hospital, and the others, succeeded despite some feeling within the Mennonite faith that mental illness was the result of having sinned—a view that moderated, in general, with the passage of time and, in partic-

---

*It was almost twenty years after the Short-Doyle Act was passed that the first of four state hospitals was "phased out" of existence, causing a great outcry; California in 1980 still had six state hospitals in operation, with a combined census, in 1979, of slightly over 8,000, with approximately as many employees as patients, and with an occupancy rate of about 93 percent. Of these six, one admits mostly retardation patients and two admit mainly "forensic" patients charged with or determined to have committed crime.

ular, with the fact that one of the church's best loved officials became mentally ill.

At the outset Kings View lent much support to California's proposed program for state support of county services, the more so because private psychiatric hospitals were eligible to contract with counties to provide the mental health services. By the mid-1960's, with state reimbursement under the Short-Doyle Act at 75 percent, Kings View started small pilot programs in three counties, itself providing the 25 percent in "matching" funds. Local interest grew slowly, but when the time came that state funds were in surplus, rapid expansion of the county programs ensued. Simultaneously the federal community mental health center program had come into being, and Kings View applied for a federal staffing grant so that it might add outpatient treatment and a consultation and education unit at Kings View Hospital. It also contracted in the early 1970's with an additional half dozen counties to provide mental health services for them. At the time of our visit in mid-1979, the Kings View Corporation was operating the county mental health programs for Madera, Mariposa, Placer, Kings, and Tulare Counties. In the way of federal funding, Kings and Tulare Counties were combined to form one catchment (service) area, and that catchment got a federal grant to expand services, then extension, so that a degree of federal financial support was available for several years.

*   *   *

The Kings County-Tulare County service area. Kings and Tulare Counties are mainly agricultural country, with rich soil and a long growing season. The "oldtimers" are characterized mainly as "conservative democrats." Nevertheless, the counties had participated in affirmative action and Headstart programs.

There are many Chicanos in the labor force and in the public schools. We were told by some that the area was "conservative in politics and fundamentalist in religion, with a streak of anti-Chicano and anti-black racism."

Visalia is Tulare County's "large town" or "small city," with about 53,000 people. Hanford, county seat of Kings County, has about 20,000 people. Fresno, with about 200,000, is the nearest city, and it is outside the mental health catchment area, as much as an hour's drive away. San Francisco and its "sophisticated" life style seem a far remove from the quiet, family-oriented folk who live in Kings and Tulare Counties, accessible only by road, passenger train, and commuter flight. We were told that in this two-county catchment area and its vicinity mental illness continued to carry a lot of stigma, which had been addressed via public service announcements on television. A Fresno TV station had also made a documentary showing a psychiatric emergency team in action. Billboards were being used to make known the mental health services locally available.

As for a locus for the inpatient services of the developing county program, there were several possibilities. Visalia had a 200-bed district hospital running a relatively low census; the small town of Tulare had a small county hospital, averaging about fifty percent occupancy; the small town of Dinuba had a 51-bed district hospital usually with a census well below capacity; and there were other quite small hospitals in Hanford, Lindsay, Exeter, and Porterville.

There was also Tulare *District* Hospital, and it was the chosen site—above all because it had, through convenient coincidence, an empty and separate unit. This district hospital, one of a type of facility specific to California and built via a bond issue, had built an extended-care facility (nursing home) which failed financially soon after two newer and more inviting nursing homes were built very close by. Tulare District Hospital thus had sitting empty a "wing," connected via passage with the main building. Kings View Corporation in 1969 signed a lease with this hospital whereby it would have the use of the empty wing while the hospital would furnish housekeeping, maintenance, food services, pharmacy and laboratory services; would include Tulare View, as the psychiatric service would be known, within its PSRO and utilization review; and would allow the psychiatric facility to bill third parties under the district hospital's provider number. The patients would be patients of Kings View Mental Health Center but subject to those rules and regulations pertaining to patients of Tulare District Hospital. In conformity with other Mennonite psychiatric facilities (Kings View, Prairie View), the psychiatric unit was dubbed Tulare View. It was fully evident, when we visited in 1979, that Tulare *District* Hospital staff in no way considered that the psychiatric service was part of that hospital, even though a corridor connected the two and a parking lot was shared. Indeed, employees of Tulare District Hospital referred to the psychiatric unit as "the other hospital."

*   *   *

In addition to 13 twin-bedded patient rooms, the unit has an entirely ample and central nursing station and some offices, a room ample for patient group meetings and indoor activities, a large dayroom with a television viewing area which also serves as the dining area, an examination room, and a medication/treatment room. Administrative offices are located across the street.

This inpatient unit is rather plain, nearly spartan, but it is clean, not cramped, and reasonably pleasant. For patients, meals

65

are brought to the unit, while most of the staff walk to the District Hospital dining room for meals.

In a separate on-site building that was formerly a laboratory, rooms of adequate quality and size offer patients a variety of social, recreational, homemaking, and craft activities. Patients surveyed indicated the most popular activities to be socializing, ceramics, grooming, yarn crafts, and Yoga.

In Tulare View's first year of operation, there were 600 admissions, and the number was rapidly increasing. Consequently, a more than usually broad emergency psychiatric service was soon created for screening (further to the screening that was done, during the day, by the outpatient clinics). It was most active from mid-afternoon onwards, and on weekends and holidays.

This emergency psychiatric program is a mobile unit serving both Tulare and Kings Counties, while operating out of Tulare View. Operating around the clock, every day of the week, the program is staffed with 12 licensed crisis workers—RN, LVN, or LPT—with one to three staff on duty each shift, depending upon the need.

With all of the participating staff well trained in dealing with psychiatric emergencies and well informed about the aspects of "crisis" presentations of would-be patients, the program had served, as was intended, not only to provide the humane consideration of readily available response but also to deal whenever practicable and feasible with the problem through outpatient service, thus eliminating the need for admission to a facility that often had an inpatient census close to capacity. Even so, by 1975 inpatient admissions had reached one thousand, and more than half of these were readmissions within one year of discharge. The reaction was to augment and amplify outpatient and day treatment in the Visalia, Porterville, Dinuba, and Tulare clinics, in an effort to reverse the trend—a goal which was so well accomplished that readmission before long had dropped from fifty percent to 15 percent of total admissions.

*   *   *

The psychiatrist directing Tulare View in 1979, Paul Mayer, had previously spent several years working in one of California's state hospitals, concurrently taking courses at the Berkeley Center for Training in Community Psychiatry. Although he was aware that several county mental health programs had collapsed, he nonetheless applied for a position at the Kings Tulare unit, and was hired, and had directed the Tulare View inpatient services since 1972. Some months before we visited, he had begun to devote about half his time to outpatient practice, since he had decided that his wide-ranging full-time inpatient responsibilities were wearing him down. It was planned for him to be succeeded by an "on board" interesting and communicative psychiatrist, James Richmond, with a diverse career pattern. After completing his residency and serving in the Navy, Richmond spent a year in private practice in Colorado, relocated to the Sacramento County mental health program and concurrently took courses at Berkeley, spent several years in private practice in Sacramento, and returned to private practice mainly with older adolescents and adults. He then "took a breather" to concentrate on his interest in and curiosity about nutrition, allergy, weight control, and chelation. Later he returned to private practice in Sacramento. In 1974 he was converted to Seventh Day Adventism. In time he saw an ad for a psychiatrist for the Tulare View unit, and he was hired about a year prior to our visit. He had been in orientation decidedly "anti-hospitalization" and had treated quite sick patients as outpatients, he said. "I don't see much point in keeping people in the hospital very long," he told us. "The hospital is an artificial place. It isolates people from the community. It grossly restricts some people who are not significantly disturbed." Thus, in Tulare View's favor for him was its short average stay, about eight days, made possible largely by thorough integration with the several outpatient clinics.

The Tulare View nursing staff was equivalent to 26 full-time employees, about one per bed. There were generally eight nursing staff by day, six in the evening, and three at night, plus six covering the week-end. There were also three social service staff and two activities staff. They were organized into two teams, one for Kings County residents, the other for Tulare County residents, each headed by one of the psychiatrists; but staff could and did rotate between the teams as needed. There was staff sufficient to provide a good range of social service, group therapy, and activity therapy. Staff seemed to be highly committed, and there was minimal turnover. All staff were salaried. The salary level was good.

Since the psychiatrists by design were present for formal admission, they could have at times a very heavy workload, but some psychiatrists in outpatient clinics thereabouts had agreed to assist by being on call some evenings and weekends. There had been no protest from local physicians about a salaried physician as unit director; there was minor complaint, however, concerning a salaried outpatient director. (An intensely negative feeling eventually developed among some physicians about Kings View Corporation, on other grounds—its ambition to develop a health maintenance organization.)

*　　*　　*

The inpatient census ranged from as few as ten up to capacity. The patients were varied. Some were chronic schizophrenics who experienced periodic exacerbations either because they stopped medication, had a life crisis, or experienced some "dietary emergency" resulting, for example, from consuming thirty cups of coffee per day. At the time we visited, one deluded young man "from the FBI" had been admitted after having stopped medication and having become a highly visible community nuisance, as he had done at previous times; having spent 19 days as an involuntary patient at Tulare View, he was slated for transfer to the state hospital, where, it was anticipated, he would be discharged after about three weeks. Another chronic psychotic patient was "psychic" and knew who had murdered whom, and where to find the bodies (but, it was added, was organized enough to keep his appointments at the welfare department). There was a woman grossly disoriented, with very high blood sugar, admitted following a seizure; a CAT scan would be made. One patient was manic depressive, well under control when medicated but periodically discontinuing medication; since admission, he screamed and frequently banged his head on the floor, and it was supposed that he would soon lose his job.

* * *

Fairly heavy medication dosages were used. Injected Prolixin was preferred for schizophrenics "because it seems to act faster and more reliably." When lithium seemed indicated for affective illness, the appropriate maintenance level was established "quickly" by means of a test dose. All patients, as soon as symptoms drop "to a level that can be tolerated in the outpatient clinic, by the family, or in a board-and-care home," were discharged. "We don't ask," we were told, "what justifies keeping him. We ask, are we justified to discharge?" It was said that problems sometimes ensued because clinics were "more oriented to psychotherapy'' and consequently reduced the level of medication. But it was often the patient who discontinued or reduced medication.

It was acknowledged that there were ''social admissions''—transients at loose ends, for example. ''When the Salvation Army closed its soup kitchen, the inpatient census went up,'' one official told us. We were also told that Tulare County had ''a great many migratory people admitted more for social and environmental reasons than because of clinical conditions; mental health has been literally the only system they can turn to.'' They were one factor in the low average stay. ''Simple alcoholics'' were not such a factor, however, since they were not admitted. If evidently merely drunk, the person was taken to jail on a charge of disorderly conduct, or to a ''social detox'' unit in the vicinity.* Those in withdrawal and evidencing the possibility of convulsion were admitted to the county hospital—as were most persons who seemed to be in poor control because of substance abuse.

Despite the heightened emphasis on clinic and day care services and other short-stay factors, the average inpatient stay had risen—from a one-time low of six-and-a-half days to eight-and-a-half. It was supposed this was mainly because, with more highly developed out-of-hospital treatment, only the ''highly disturbed'' were being admitted. Most of the patients had relatives who visited, and the visiting hours are generous. There was no formal limit on stay, and an occasional patient, when it seemed justified, had stayed for a month or more. However, thirty percent were ''crisis admits'' staying less than 48 hours.

---

*This facility, Hamilton House, or, formally, the Tulare County Substance Abuse Program, is also operated by Kings View, and the funds for it come primarily through a subcontract that Kings View has with Tulare County.

(An additional group, mostly overnight emergencies who came in voluntarily, were on site less than 24 hours, and therefore not included in inpatient statistics.)

If the improved patient had come from a home that would take him back, he returned to it. Otherwise, he could be transferred to a board-and-care facility, if that would serve and if a bed were available. Next down the line were the "L-facilities," a euphemism for California's privately owned, usually small, and usually programless locked psychiatric facilities, of which there were two within fifty miles of Tulare. From our own sole exposure to an "L-facility," elsewhere in the state, it was hard to imagine who could not be "managed" there, but we were told that some cannot, and the sole remaining "resource" is the state hospital—in this case, since a nearer one had been closed, Napa State Hospital, more than two hundred miles away, with almost 2,000 beds and an average occupancy of 96 percent.

*   *   *

We talked with a one-time mental health center psychiatrist who had gone into private practice in Visalia. He thought the psychological separateness of side-by-side Tulare District Hospital and Tulare View had proved more useful than harmful. Inevitably there had been "unfortunate incidents"—specifically, some "escapes," which were upsetting to the community and the District Hospital board. It seemed clear that there was no yearning on the part of Tulare View staff to be "further integrated" or "more identified" with Tulare District Hospital.

The future, expectably, was uncertain. Tulare View could likely continue its relationship with Tulare District Hospital, of whose staff Tulare View physicians were necessarily, if largely *pro forma,* members. Payment by Tulare View to Tulare District was on a "cost reimbursement" basis so that it could not make a profit. Tulare District was, of record, responsible for the quality of care at Tulare View.

In Visalia, at a newer, more ambiant 224-bed district hospital with an average census of 68 percent, there was no psychiatric service. One was wanted; the Health Service Agency for that part of California would not approve it, however, even though Visalia had the larger population and was a 15 minute drive from Tulare. It was conceivable even, that both Kings and Tulare Counties would in time decline to contract any longer for inpatient psychiatric care, even though California law requires that patients be given 14 days of "local" treatment before being transferred to a state hospital. (In some parts of the state, the state hospital itself, when reasonably at hand, had been contracted with as provider of the 14-day "local" treatment. But Napa, the state hospital serving Kings and Tulare Counties, being two hundred miles away, would find it impracticable to provide "local" treatment.)

One influential executive at Kings View Corporation asserted that "psychiatry in a general hospital is a big pain in the neck. The pertinent rules and regulations are too different. The general hospital setting isn't appropriate for day care or recreational therapy. Furthermore, if the census is lower in the medical service, inevitably the psychiatric service is stuck with disproportionately high charges for meals and everything else."

In the meantime, all staff vacancies at Tulare View were "frozen" in the face of California's Proposition 13.

*   *   *

On balance, nonetheless, this inpatient service seemed well organized and efficient, with generally high morale. The unit would probably benefit if the psychiatrists had more time for staff education and staff interaction. It would probably benefit too, if the four clinics had some systematic means of letting the inpatient staff know the status of formerly hospitalized patients being followed by the clinics.

For the record, none of the federal community mental health center grants had been available for this inpatient operation, whose support money had come mainly from the state's mental health program and from MediCal, California's version of Medicaid, and Medicare.

With the closing and potential further closings of state hospitals, it seemed likely that more and more chronic mental patients would be "emerging" within communities and that a number of them would require brief hospitalization during periodic crises; the Tulare View/Tulare District relationship was an arrangement with the potential for making local psychiatric inpatient care available in low-population-density settings with limited resources and a limited need for inpatient treatment. The attachment allowed third-party billing without requiring that the psychiatric unit be heavily dependent on the general hospital. At the same time, it perpetuated the gap between psychiatric and other medical practice, as suggested by the fact that in the year prior to our visit only two psychiatric patients had been admitted to Tulare View directly by psychiatrists in private practice.

*   *   *

We were impressed with many major components of this service and pondered how recently the time was that one with emotional illness could hardly have anticipated the availability of so well-staffed and readily accessible a service as this one. Its being there was, like so many things in life, the product of curious coincidences—the interest of the Kings View parent operation, the availability of a quite adequate and vacant building, and the advent of a time when, increasingly, well-trained staff wanted to get to a small-town setting, away from the stresses of metropolitan living. If in a sense Tulare View was a distinctly separate operation from Tulare District Hospital, in a sense it was not, and despite the separate governing auspices, psychiatry was perhaps as much a part of the range of services on this small "campus" as were the other specialized services of Tulare District. We were in pursuit of small-hospital psychiatric services that seemed to have done well, and this program, we felt, fully met our expectations.

Subsequently

Reduced funds as a result of Proposition 13 and the ending of federal staffing support had taken its toll. With the expiration of the federal staffing grant, Kings-Tulare Community Mental Health Center was separated into the Kings View Mental Health Services for Tulare County and the Kings View Mental Health Services for Kings County, while Tulare View continued to provide inpatient services to both counties. There was at Tulare View by the end of 1981 no longer a full-time psychiatrist; Dr. Mayer continued as medical director and the psychiatrists from the four counseling centers reported to Tulare View daily to follow patients from their service areas. Only one nursing position had been lost, but with only a half-time social worker many of the functions of the social service department had been assumed by the nursing staff. The activities department had but one salaried (and trained) worker, assisted by numerous volunteers from the community.

The psychiatric emergency team had been reduced to five licensed workers and provided limited services only to Tulare County—to walk-ins, via telephone and by outcall, after regular working hours. Weekdays, from 8:00 to 5:00, the emergency services were provided by the four counseling centers.

Recreational and craft activities had been relocated to more satisfactory quarters in the basement of Tulare View.

Kings View no longer contracted with Tulare County to provide alcohol detoxification; the funds were now allocated to two existing long-term halfway houses, one in Visalia, the other in Porterville.

Memorial Hospital of South Amboy, New Jersey

SOUTH AMBOY MEMORIAL Hospital was established, with fifty beds, just after World War I, and it was named to memorialize the casualties of a war-related munitions explosion. It is in a town whose individual population figure in some respects hardly matters, since the town is towards the southern end of an industrial, transportation, and residential sprawl that extends almost uninterruptedly for 25 miles northward to Newark and Jersey City. It is just across the Raritan River from Perth Amboy.

South Amboy is one of a number of townships thereabouts descendent from farming communities established three centuries ago. By way of commuter train, it is an hour and a world away from Manhattan. The voluntary Memorial Hospital, now with 144 beds and an average occupancy of 71 percent, provides an intensive care unit, a pediatrics unit, diagnostic and laboratory facilities that are thoroughly and modernly equipped, a 24-hour emergency room, and well-equipped medical and surgical wards.

Built with funds that came partly from the federal mental health centers program is a 15-bed psychiatric unit and its adjacent psychiatric day program. They are subject to the hospital's rules and regulations, bill under its provider number, and are included in its PSRO and utilization reviews. A few minutes away, across the river, is the much larger—480 bed—Perth Amboy general hospital, with psychiatric inpatient, outpatient, emergency, and consultation and education services. Any other general hospital psychiatric services are in towns closer to New York City than to South Amboy. Most local folk are inclined to use South Amboy Memorial for all the hospital services they need and which it has available. It does not provide, for example, a burn unit, but patients requiring special services not provided here can be transported, if necessary by helicopter (the hospital having its own helipad) to a hospital that does.

Inpatient psychiatric services are additionally available at two fairly close and fairly long-stay private psychiatric hospitals that usually have waiting lists, and do not have emergency rooms.

All of the staff of the mental health services within the South Amboy hospital are in fact employees of the hospital itself, which writes their paychecks. The federal mental health staffing grant, when we visited, was all the way down to the 25 percent level, and soon to expire.

The hospital was, thus, the main locus of a mental health center, providing *a*) the emergency service, *b*) one outpatient clinic,*c*) inpatient care, and *d*) rehabilitation care, which combines day care as such and posthospital aftercare. On the hospital's attending staff there were no psychiatrists, mainly, we were told, because psychiatrists in private practice thereabouts were said to prefer not to do inpatient work because many persons living in the area could not afford the cost; many of the hospital's patients are indigent. Northwards, nearer to New York

---

*Additional outpatient care was provided by the East Brunswick Guidance Clinic, which maintained separate records and is located nine miles from the hospital.

78

City, some private practice psychiatrists liked to do inpatient work, it being possible for them to do adequately well financially through patient rounds and ECT treatments.

In earlier years, we were told, Middlesex County residents had either to go some distance for psychiatric care in a general hospital, or gain admission to one of the private psychiatric hospitals, or become patients at the state mental hospital in Marlboro, about 15 miles away. With about 900 beds, Marlboro State Hospital had in the late 1970's an average occupancy of about seventy percent. All involuntary patients are required, by law, to be taken there, since New Jersey law will not permit involuntary psychiatric admission to general hospitals. In New Jersey, health care is expectably under the Department of Health, except that mental health only is under the Department of Human Services.

*　　*　　*

Construction of the inpatient facilities at Memorial Hospital was completed in 1974, with construction financed partly by a federal construction grant—without the help of which a psychiatric unit would probably not have been developed. It consisted of 15 beds in semiprivate rooms, plus three "holding beds" used for patients thought to require from 24 to 48 hours of observation for evaluation purposes prior to regular admission; most of these were persons intoxicated when brought in who, after sobering up, signed themselves out. The unit is located on the fourth floor of a new wing and near to the medical-surgical units. It was designed much like other such services, with an open nursing station, a moderately large occupational therapy area, several small lounges for group discussions and relaxing, and a dining area.

Its early history was one of borderline tumult, with the inpatient program considered "less than viable" and with little liaison with either the rest of the hospital or with the community.

Late in 1976 there came to the staff a young psychiatrist named Richard Cassone, who took hold and provided clear leadership and imparted a sense of direction. At the time of our visit the service operated at or near capacity much of the time. Half or more of the patients had a primary alcoholism diagnosis, and while they were roomed together with other psychiatric patients they had a separate treatment program.

Admissions came primarily through the hospital's sole and all-purpose emergency service, which putatively could hold for observation a person seemingly emotionally disturbed but in practice rarely did so. Rather, the psychiatric unit was telephoned, and a staff member, designated a counselor and required to be a college graduate, responded, made a preliminary determination whether the person was appropriate for inpatient admission either as alcoholic or for other psychiatric indications and if so called for Dr. Cassone or his associate to come down; at night or on days when the psychiatrists were not on duty, the emergency room physician and the aide conferred, the physician serving mainly to "clear the patient medically." If admission on psychiatric grounds seemed indicated, the psychiatrist on call was contacted, and, in most instances, gave authorization via telephone for admission.

Patients referred from the outpatient clinics or by the center's transitional services unit could be admitted to the inpatient service directly (that is, bypassing the emergency room) and such admissions represented about twenty percent of the total.

Dr. Cassone or his fellow psychiatrist, Dr. Nina Sachinvala, promptly—on day of admission or, in the case of a prior nighttime or weekend admission, during the next day of duty—took a medical history, did a physical examination and a psychiatric evaluation on all admissions, and assigned the new patient to one of the counselors. (The policy of having the psychiatrist do the physical examination had been one factor, evidently a large one, in the resignation of some of the psychiatrists who preceded Cassone and Sachinvala.)

*   *   *

The staff. Altogether there were usually 25 mental health employees, a number of whom had been on hand for several years. "For the most part," the nursing supervisor told us, "we're a distinct service. When we have problems here, we don't run to the nursing service with them." This nurse supervisor hired her own employees and she provided their orientation. Most were, at time of hiring, already working elsewhere within the hospital and requested to be transferred to the psychiatric unit. By day there were five nurses, two licensed practical nurses, and one mental health counselor; on the evening shift, four nurses and two counselors; and at night, three nurses and one counselor.

The counselors have a germane bachelor's degree, and most are pursuing a master's degree. Under the supervision of a doctoral candidate in psychology, they rotate shifts, are available 24 hours a day, function via schedule to cover the emergency room, and cover a telephone crisis line.

Dr. Cassone was "center-wide" *medical* director (the mental health center director was a psychologist); Dr. Sachinvala, more specifically and less broadly, was director of inpatient services, and there was a vacant position for a third psychiatrist, to head up the transitional, day, and consultation programs.

Dr. Cassone impressed us as an intelligent man who was well trained and who before coming to the South Amboy hospital had contemplated with some care what kind of practice and what kind of setting would be right for him. He did his psychiatric training at St. Vincent's Hospital in New York City, then did his military service, and after discharge spent "three unsatisfying months" at a psychiatric hospital he felt was more concerned with making a profit than with quality of care. In the classified columns of *Psychiatric News* he saw the South Amboy job advertised, and applied for it. "They let me do things much the way I think best," he said, and he added that "the staff is very good." His experience with community mental health at the time we talked with him totaled two-and-a-half years, and his feelings about it were mixed. He felt that the bureaucratic constraints interfered with the ability to provide service. He said that the majority of patients live near the hospital, and he had the impression that there were few from the southern part of the center's "catchment area," partly because the availability of the services was not well known there and partly because of transportation difficulties. Consequently, there were plans afoot to develop services there.

Dr. Cassone had spent most of his life in big cities, and he felt that in smaller places political considerations loomed larger, or at least were a more discernible factor in clinical matters. He thought that variety was one reason that he found his work satisfying, with a combination of administrative and clinical responsibilities and doing consultations on patients on medical wards, plus some industrial consultations. He was seeing private patients three evenings a week, although he was not permitted to see those who lived in that county, unless they called him direct, and furthermore, he could not have his private practice office in that county. Seeing private practice patients all day long, he thought, would exceed his tolerance. With private patients he sometimes used hypnosis and behavior modification principles. We were not surprised to learn that the first higher education of this articulate man had been in theology and philosophy.

Dr. Sachinvala, trained in India, told us that she thought that "most of our admissions are quite justifiable. Occasionally we find we've been stuck with someone who has 'learned the technique,' but most admissions are really necessary. As soon as the crisis is over, we discharge them. We emphasize getting the family in and giving them support and teaching them how to cope with the circumstances, so they feel better, and most of the time they will take the patient back." When we asked her, she told us that she thought there are many Americans who turn to hospitals when a crisis occurs "because they have no support system." In other countries, she added, there are more often relatives standing by to help family members until stabilization sets in after a loss or some other crisis. "Here many people are alone. Half the time even relatives don't want to have anything to do with each other. People have become too independent and too much into moneymaking and have ignored many social aspects of life. Socialization is often superficial, with little feeling and little warmth."

*   *   *

The treatment program—psychiatry. Mental health inpatients spent their days in individual sessions with their designated counselors, in a variety of group therapy sessions that had a feeling of openness and task orientation, and in a variety of occupational and recreational activities run jointly by the inpatient and day program staff. Psychoactive medication was prescribed for most patients—about eighty percent. Prior to discharge, inpatients were given referrals to the outpatient clinics, or were transferred to the day or transitional programs. The average inpatient stay was eight days—not pulled down artificially by the large number of alcoholism admissions, since such patients who leave within 48 hours of admission were not counted as having been admitted.

The treatment approach was seen as a "case management system" akin to the Balanced Service System elucidated by Dr. Donald Miles. The family involvement which Dr. Sachinvala mentioned was not only encouraged but was sometimes made a prerequisite for continuation of hospital stay.

Some of the inpatients participate in the day program. Its director, a doctoral candidate in psychology, had urged combining the day and the transitional programs. He told us he was glad that the day program was scheduled to be relocated, because he felt that psychiatric day programs should not take place within hospitals. In the interim, staff took patients out of the hospital for activities most days, to the YMCA and to the old house across the street where the transitional program for chronic patients was quartered and where as many as 14 persons at a time cooked, sewed, and did like things. The patients moved easily between these components; some inpatients participated in the day program, and some transitional patients living in the community participated in the day program for chronic patients, called Horizons. (It was, for a time, limited to those discharged from hospital.) It operated Monday through Wednesday and on Friday from 9:00 to 3:00 and on Thursday from 1:00 to 9:00 p.m., transportation was provided for those who needed it, and various patients were scheduled to attend from as little as one up to five days per week. But the inpatients could readily "cross the street" to the old house, and consequently at times the "inpatients" and the "day patients" of the inhospital day program were mainly one and the same group.

*   *   *

The treatment program—alcoholism. The program for alcoholism patients did not differ greatly in content from that for other patients but it was run mainly by staff especially informed about alcoholics—either by having been one, or through having taken special training, or both. There were three alcoholism counselors. There were scheduled activities seven days a week. One of the counselors, a recovered alcoholic who took courses at the well-known training program at Rutgers University, told us "there are a couple of people who are in and out with such frequency that it seems they think the hospital is a hotel. Anyway, they are willing to come back here because they are treated like decent human beings. With first admissions we sometimes find after they're sober that they're schizophrenic, since alcohol masks that and some other psychotic states." She showed us the 26-question form they had developed and used as a kind of "status indicator." Those first admissions willing to do so could stay as long as two weeks, with the county paying sixty percent and the hospital, if necessary, absorbing the rest of the cost. With readmissions, the staff decided, after five days, whether the patient seemed motivated enough to justify continued treatment. People who had sobered up and didn't want to stay were released but were told they could come back for the aftercare program. They were given a packet of information about Alcoholics Anonymous, Alateen, and Al-Anon, all of which were active in the vicinity; also, the unit itself provided aftercare counseling for patient and family jointly. This group met on Saturdays for what was called group therapy; for individual therapy and medication, as needed, by Dr. Cassone; and all who attended were required to be sober.

Cassone told us that "a lot of our alcoholism admissions are quite sick physically and badly need treatment for several days." But if a person brought to the emergency room appeared to be "merely drunk" he can be held, on the psychiatric unit, "to keep him off the road." (It is New Jersey's alcohol rehabilitation treatment act that allows a patient to be held for as long as 48 hours without being admitted.)

We were told that alcoholism admissions were "of all ages—

85

from 15 to elderly,'' usually in trouble with their families or at their jobs, mentally confused and not knowing why. "Many," one counselor told us, "think nobody cares about them. They feel hopeless and helpless. Their self-esteem is low, they're insecure and feel inadequate. A minority, however, are, or act, arrogant, grandiose, and egotistical."

The administrative offices of the mental health center, located in space adjacent to the psychiatric unit, were slated to move to a new building, after which time, Cassone hoped, it would be possible to use the vacated space for alcohol detoxification, since there was no specific place, at the time we visited, for patients needing to be withdrawn under supervision, and they represented a large portion of admissions to psychiatry. "Once they're medically clear," he said, "we could send them to the neighboring area where they could be treated at less expense and with limited need for medical involvement."

*   *   *

About 98 percent of inpatients live within the county. Diagnostically, 83 percent fall into three categories: alcohol disorders, schizophrenia, and major affective disorders. The remaining 17 percent are spread among a dozen other diagnoses.

During our visit, a patient, a college student, was brought in by the police, who had picked him up on a highway nearby, where, after his car ran out of gasoline, he was attempting to demolish it. He struck out wildly at the police. When he saw us at the inpatient unit, he asked whether we might be lawyers because "I need my rights protected." He was clearly out of control but clearly evidenced a desire to regain control. Momentarily ashamed of having intentionally damaged a light fixture, he soon resumed pacing and lashing out. His parents, in a distant state, had been called. The psychiatrist who examined him was attuned to the possibility of drug psychosis but thought it more likely that the young man was in a psychotic state that had not needed any help from drug abuse. She wanted to hold him until it could be arranged for him to be returned to a hospital in his home town, but it seemed clear that he posed too much risk to the ward, and so it was arranged, as New Jersey law requires in the case of involuntary patients, for him to be transported to the not-distant state hospital. Within two hours of his arrival with the policemen, he was transferred; there seemed little question that he would be difficult to manage and was potentially dangerous, and evidently strong. (The unit at Memorial Hospital had no seclusion room and also it had windows that opened, by design, and doors not locked, by policy.) It was saddening to accept that there was no alternative but to transfer him to safer facilities.

* * *

Intrahospital consultation. Said the hospital administrator, "The great need and the great potential for psychiatric input on medical wards lies in such situations as the vasectomy patient or the family of the patient with terminal cancer." That Cassone was performing well in consultations of such nature was evident, the administrator told us, from what was said in the meetings of various hospital committees.

* * *

Bureaucratism. Although New Jersey regulations will not permit the admission, even to general hospitals *willing* to accept them, of involuntary patients to psychiatric units, it simultaneously requires that South Amboy Memorial and similar hospitals *screen* all of the patients presented on emotional bases. This is perhaps mainly because the psychiatric hospitals to which they

87

may be involuntarily committed do not have emergency rooms.

The future. There was some happy anticipation of the day when what was called by the hospital administrator "an entire health village" would be completed. Its development was under way at the time of our visit. It would provide acute care and many other things. "It will be total," we were told. To be built on 15 acres of donated land three miles away, its interior would have 120,000 square feet. One specific intention was to arrange with large corporations in the vicinity to provide to their employees alcohol education programs, which, it was hoped, would reduce the incidence of diminished performance and outright dysfunction from the heavy and sustained drinking which many of the citizenry engage in—just as we had heard at the other places we visited.

Finale. The reader will have perceived that the authors were persuaded that this was a quality service, with responsible and well-trained staff, and an enthusiastic hospital administrator who wanted things done and could get them done. The psychiatry service and its affiliated programs were, in the most positive sense of the word, a resource for the community.

Subsequently

By 1982 a number of developments had occurred. The inpatient staff had been expanded to eight registered nurses, an LPN, and fourteen inpatient counselors. The counselors, Dr. Cassone advised, take full part in treatment planning, case management, and liaison duties, in conjunction with the psychiatrist who replaced Dr. Sachinvala, after she departed to study forensic psychiatry. The counselors, in Dr. Cassone's words, "are all-purpose people." He felt that "the quality of the staff. has easily doubled" since our visit in 1979.

The psychiatric day program had relocated to its own building, two miles south of hospital, and was serving over 150 clients. An affiliation had been established with a privately funded agency which provides housing for psychiatric patients, and there were 18 center clients living on their own and caring for their needs with the support of the day program.

Two outreach centers had been set up in the southern part of the service area, each providing individual counseling and making home visits—which include family therapy within the patient's home as needed.

Industrial consultations had increased, with the center having entered into three contracts with local corporations for weekly visits from the staff.

An additional psychiatrist had been hired, half time, to work with the Horizon Program.

The three alcohol counselors had been placed under supervision of the inpatient counselor supervisor and thus had an increased amount of supervision and more involvement in case management.

An adolescent day school had been started, providing service for 15 students considered emotionally disturbed. A psychiatrist was spending ten hours per week providing evaluation, counseling, and medication.

An Early Intervention Program was started with offices *a)* in the hospital, *b)* in the former day hospital premises, and *c)* at the two satellite outreach centers, and was providing individual and family therapy—here again, in the patient's home when necessary.

Memorial Hospital
Tampa, Florida

MEMORIAL HOSPITAL, an attractive 140-bed proprietary hospital, built in 1970 and located conveniently in a good section of Tampa, has had several chapters in a short history. It was designed to be divided between an inpatient kidney dialysis program and a nursing home.

Very shortly, by 1971, the floor designated for a nursing home was converted to a psychiatric inpatient service, initially headed by a full-time salaried psychiatrist director and intended to provide inhospital treatment to patients who would be referred by the numerous local psychiatrists in private practice. These psychiatrists declined, however, to refer patients, and few of them did so. Consequently, it was not long before the position of salaried staff psychiatrist was abolished, and it was arranged that the local psychiatrists in private individual or group practice would become an attending staff.

For a time, the 46-bed psychiatric unit ran a high census and a high ratio of staff to patient. It operated as a type of milieu approach with nurses, social workers, occupational therapists, and "milieu workers" grouped in teams, with each patient designated as the responsibility of one of the particular teams.

The hospital was subsequently purchased by an out-of-state firm that both owned and operated several general hospitals, none of which had a psychiatric service. Its executive staff surveyed Memorial Hospital and decided that the staff of the psychiatry service could be reduced, considerably, and simultaneously took unto itself the right of hiring staff, which theretofore had been the prerogative of the attending psychiatrists. Both decisions sat far from well with them, and since inpatient psychiatric beds were sufficiently available at other hospitals in the area, the psychiatric census at Memorial soon dropped from near-capacity to three patients. Given the advantage of hindsight, it seemed notable that a corporation owning half a dozen hospitals would so rapidly and radically alter a thriving unit as soon to render it virtually unused.

The new ownership capitulated by means of replacing the administrator, transferring there as replacement the administrator of another of its hospitals. This young man, relatively newly arrived when we visited the facility in 1979, was clearly bright, alert, assertive, and accommodating. He had not previously worked in a hospital with a psychiatric unit, but whatever he needed to know he had quickly learned since his arrival about 18 months before our visit. The inpatient staff, even though smaller than it had been in the "thriving years," had been augmented. That the psychiatrists were of significance was made clear to them; their hiring rights were restored, and by ones and twos they resumed admitting patients to Memorial. Playing a constructive role throughout these ups and downs was Holly Gray, director of nursing, who had "stuck to her last."

When the hospital first opened, the psychiatry service had occupied the entire top (fourth) floor. When the census fell greatly, the section towards one end of the floor was "deleted" and its subsequent use was, at the time of our visit, still to be determined. Consequently, what we saw in 1979 was a 26-bed unit with ample ancillary and support space. It was at high census, as was often the case, and while there were some who wished to see the deleted twenty beds restored, others were content to have the unit remain at 26. In any case, the attractive facility was regaining its "top of line" image.

The entry door to the unit is locked at all times, a practice that seemed to be satisfactory to staff and, with rare exceptions, the patients. There were usually adolescent patients, some of whom might simply "walk away," and occasional court-referred patients, but even apart from these considerations, we were told, most of the patients preferred the sense of privacy which a locked unit afforded, so that the matter seemed a combination of "locking in" patients while "locking out" others so as to provide privacy.

Within a few feet of the entry, the unit opens up onto a quite large, extremely attractive, and comfortably and tastefully furnished "common room." One portion has tables and chairs where patients and most of the staff take their meals. The nursing station is of good size, open, and accessible. A small kitchen unit has a constant supply of coffee, fresh fruit, and some other foods. There is an activity room, used mainly as and well equipped for arts and crafts; it is of moderate size, large enough to accommodate eight or ten patients at one time. There is another room, untitled, moderately large, furnished like a living room, quite suitable for a variety of meetings and activities for about a dozen patients at a time. The unit, we felt, was as appropriately designed and attractively furnished as any we have seen in any general hospital. It is functional and at the same time has what one observer called "a marvelously warm feeling—of a home, a college dorm, and a camp all combined into one." The sole "security room," having internal corners with sharp edges, could not be used for an agitated or combative person.

The staff readily acknowledged that the unit declined to admit aggressive patients. The vast majority of patients were voluntarily admitted—by or on referral from one of the 15 psychiatrists on the attending staff—and, in most cases, had private health insurance covering substantially all expenses. There were few black patients, not because of any policy of limiting their number, but as the result of a variety of social and financial factors. Worth noting was that the hospital had no emergency room, let alone an emergency service specific to psychiatry, so that patients could be admitted only when referred by an attending psychiatrist or, occasionally, when someone by chance "self presented" and an attending could be contacted to serve to admit him.

* * *

The staff. We found it interesting that this comparatively "opulent" facility should have a lower staff-to-patient ratio than certain more run-of-the-mill physical facilities we had visited: here, the equivalent of twenty staff (plus the attending psychiatrists who made daily rounds) for a capacity census of 26. The previously mentioned director of nursing, who had had children before completing nursing training, which included a sequence at a psychiatric clinic, joined the Memorial Hospital staff about two years after the psychiatric service opened. It seemed a matter both of her personality and of the allegiance of having stuck with the unit that accounted for her clearly strong influence, which she seemed to use simultaneously in the service of the patients, the psychiatrists, and the unit staff. She was enfranchised to hire and, as necessary, train nursing staff. The unit had seven registered nurses, three with psychiatric training; one

LPN; three attendants called milieu workers; two aides; a school teacher; an occupational therapist; a social worker; and a unit clerk. The milieu workers, required to have a college degree, could "counsel" whereas aides could not, but the distinction between how much and what they did with patients and how they did it was unclear. There was no organized, formal, and scheduled inservice training; beyond orientation, training seemed to be via preceptor and "through doing."

The chief social worker was also the sole social worker, and she had been on the job less than a week when we visited. The daughter of an attending psychiatrist, she had come to Memorial from a private psychiatric facility in the vicinity. She anticipated that other social workers would be recruited to serve on her staff. Perhaps because few of the patients had such elemental traditional social service problems as lack of a place to live or attaining eligibility for public assistance, she focused mostly on "therapeutic interactions," which might well prove useful, since patient involvement individually with formally trained therapists was limited to the daily rounds of attending psychiatrists. It was not clear whether she and her staff-to-come would work therapeutically with families. We found some of the persuasions she put forth to be interesting—particularly that it is not uncommon for the "patient" to have made a choice, at least semiconsciously, to become a hospitalizable psychiatric case as a means of avoiding or evading other pain—stress—and that it was not infrequent for a patient to be a recently divorced woman who required hospitalization "because she hasn't learned that it is normal to live single." She thought the average stay, longer than in many general hospital psychiatry services, was too short for many patients—the many "who somehow didn't learn how to cope with stress" and could not learn in a three-week stay. By hospital policy, discharged patients were entitled to four subsequent social work visits, in an attempt to give newly discharged patients support. "Frequently," we were told, "ex–patients call back to the unit to tell the staff about accomplishments as well as periods of feeling low."

The activities therapist—the only one, in contrast with a one-time department of seven—did not have formal credentials (such as Occupational Therapist Registered), but she seemed a solid, forthright, competent, and responsible person who had a sensible understanding of what it is realistic to hope to accomplish through such work with patients, and her main regret appeared to be that the physical space did not allow a larger number to participate at a given time. It seemed likely she would be accorded at least one fellow worker, which she needed.

* * *

The patients. We were unable to review any records because of regulations about confidentiality. While there were sometimes elderly patients and teenagers, the modal group, when we visited, were in the range of post-high school up to the early thirties. Several looked to be heavily medicated. Few seemed agitated or otherwise externally evidenced disturbance. The most frequent cause of admission was depression, with a predominance of women of middle age. Schizophrenia was next most frequent. Third were adolescents of varied diagnoses. Heavy drinkers, unless the drinking seemed definitely to be one among several symptoms of major disorder, were admitted to an adjacent but separate five-bed "detoxification program" (although at admission point, not all were toxic).

The average stay of 21 days probably resulted mainly from philosophy. Through implicit and explicit screening, those usually brief-term alcoholic "dry outs" and those brief-term chronic patients accepted in anticipation of early transfer were not for-

mally admitted. Few patients cooperative at admission became
so unmanageable as to necessitate transfer.

*   *   *

The program. There were various things for patients to do—
but not enough, in the opinion of staff. While the range was
good, including "interpersonal" group therapy, art groups *cum*
expressive discussion of the art work, and an admirable and
suitably individual educational program for adolescents, a patient could not participate unless his physician consented, and,
even if he did, participation was not mandatory. In the after-
noons patients went on walks. Evenings they played Ping Pong
or various card or other games.

Many were visited by relatives; most patients came "from
home" and returned home, although a divorce in process or of
recent occurrence was not an uncommon factor. If the census
was high, more than one each of social worker and activities
therapist was needed; if there were many adolescents, more than
one teacher could prove useful, since schoolwork was individual. The money to build and the place to put a greenhouse had
been settled upon. A gym and swimming pool were wished for.
Clearly more space for outdoor recreation would be helpful—
and so would a quiet room on the unit.

Deserving particular note was the program of the "milieu
worker" school teacher. This young man had taught briefly in
public school, had had slight exposure to "special ed," had
decided to cram for graduate school, and needed a part-time job.
He came to Memorial Hospital by chance and became the teacher
in psychiatry by chance—seemingly a very lucky chance for the
unit. He had accomplished much with the teenagers, who, said
other staff, "are frustrating and hard on the nerves, and depress-
ing in that they waste their lives on drugs." This teacher was not

97

doing "special education," he said. "These children have no learning disabilities, and most are unusually bright and open. They don't see themselves as sick but as being punished by parents who, they say, 'kicked me out.' " But he was inclined, despite their self-assessment, to feel that some were definitely disturbed—usually on the road to full-blown sociopathy. Some, he thought, were unlikely ever to change until they burn out, whereas others "used the con knowingly" as a means of testing. He saw the parents as varied—some quite "together," some "as out-of-shape or more so" than the youngster. This man, who said he had "come from the sticks," was bright, integrated, and an expert at dealing in a straightforward way with these young patients. Since all three of the law schools he had applied to had accepted him, he would soon be leaving—seemingly to the unit's loss.

* * *

The psychiatrists. There were 15 attending psychiatrists; one or another, changing from time to time, who was willing to serve as chief, was so designated by his fellow attendings, and was compensated for his time equivalent to about one day per week. We saw the majority of attendings in assembly, as our first Tampa activity, at a monthly breakfast at which they plus certain staff gather. This event consisted partly of amiable conversation but mainly of a lengthy case presentation, followed by discussion. Pro forma business matters were also dealt with.

Those of the psychiatrists with whom we later had individual interviews were all well informed, obviously attentive to their patients, and considerate of the staff. They consistently required that nursing notes be of high quality, and they paid careful attention to laboratory studies. They frequently prescribed medication and stated that other attendings did also and estimated that psychotropics were used with about ninety percent of patients. Individual therapy was also widely used, but mainly back in the office, after discharge. Some of the attendings used family therapy if it seemed indicated.

These things seemed clear: *a*) comparatively, the supply of inpatient psychiatric beds in the area was generous, and, for the population of the market area, so was the supply of private-practice psychiatrists; *b*) nonetheless, the demand for service, including hospitalization, was high. The psychiatrists seemed well thought of by other professions, and they had considerable say in how the facilities they utilized were organized and run.

*   *   *

Finances. At a census that had recently averaged about 75 percent, the unit was comfortably solvent, at a daily rate no higher than at much less attractive and comfortable facilities. The rate included all services except physician visits and medications; if the numbers of ancillary staff were increased, as was variously discussed, the hospital's charge would necessarily be somewhat higher. The administrator emphasized, as those elsewhere did, that the psychiatric unit, even with a room rate higher than in medical wards, "is no gold mine," because psychiatry generated little of the additional revenue of medical-surgical units. To keep this service at high quality while keeping its cost equivalent to other services called for common cause between administration and attending staff.

Miscellany and conclusions. It is our practice, when that is possible, to consider facilities for what they are rather than what they are not. This unit, since it lacked safely secure facilities, could not accept significantly "acting up" or aggressive patients; it could accept only those who could pay themselves or through insurance or other third-party access; since the hospital was proprietary, it was expected to yield some return on the capital invested in it. For those who could arrange to pay, to accept that they should be in a hospital, and to conform by and large to reasonable rules and restrictions, this unit seemed better than most we have visited. It was entirely one version of ''the medical model,'' with the physician clearly in charge. Apparently it did not occur to anyone thereabout to challenge this approach, nor did we see that it should be challenged, given that the psychiatrists were of evident good quality and were conscientious. We did not find it surprising to hear that ''some patients don't want to leave, because they're living better here than in the community—particularly those older folks who haven't been touched or hugged or loved in years.'' Whether the distress of divorce or conflict with parents constitutes grounds for hospitalization depends on the individual's total situation and is a problem for—as it doubtless is to—utilization review committees.

Subsequently

By 1982 the hospital had again changed hands, having been bought by another chain, and it had been expanded to a 174-bed facility. The vacant beds on the psychiatric floor had been converted in part to an alcohol detoxification unit (eight beds) and the remaining 12 beds were used for overflow from the medical-surgical units.

The psychiatry staff had been expanded slightly, with a man experienced in arts and activities assigned, full time, to the afternoon and evening hours, and with a part-time social worker who three mornings a week led adult groups.

The departed school teacher was replaced by another, who also functioned as milieu worker; the school sessions were reduced to an hour and a half three mornings a week, with outings taking place on two other mornings.

The director of psychiatric nursing, departed for health reasons, was replaced by a "head nurse/manager," and there were four other full-time registered nurses, three part-time registered nurses, an LPN, an aide, three milieu workers full-time and two part time, and a ward clerk. With coverage based on census, the nursing hours allotted per patient averaged 3.9 per 24 hours.

The aspiration for a greenhouse having been put aside, regular hours were now scheduled at the Jewish Community Center for patient use of gym and swimming pool. And an ex-patient came to the hospital ward regularly each week to lead an activities therapy class.

Chelsea Community Hospital
Chelsea, Michigan

W HAT HAD BEEN operating since the early 1970's as a community hospital in the small Michigan town of Chelsea had its beginning as a nursing home, built in the 1960's by a doctor whose intent from the outset was to convert the facility into a general hospital. The visitor who comes to what evolved into Chelsea Community Hospital drives into attractive grounds, where there are an abundance of trees, an abundance of parking, and attractive low-set buildings with a total of 116 beds. The 51-bed "east" unit, undifferentiated even by a direction sign from the rest of the aggregation, had accommodations for 16 patients in a psychiatry unit, for a dozen more in a highly autonomous substance abuse (chiefly alcoholism) program, and for 23 more in a general medical service.

This and the abutting building are attractive. The staff, the attending physicians, and others working in the east unit, however, were dissatisfied with the amount of lounge facilities and other common areas for patients, feeling that, since considerable of bed capacity had been converted into units for psychiatric and substance abuse patients, proportionately more common area was needed; but even if less than adequate in expanse, the facilities were available, and they were inviting. Patients were accommodated in attractive and pleasant semiprivate rooms. There is a tranquility about the outlook and about the atmosphere. If one must be hospitalized for psychiatric reason, the psychiatric section at this small hospital is a more attractive place than most that we have seen.

The reputation of the hospital in the community and surrounding area was said to be good, with the hospital viewed as a better place in which to be a patient than some other hospitals thereabouts, what with the facility not only closer at hand but also more attractive. Chelsea Community Hospital's general reputation, it was felt, was helped by its having, despite its relatively small size, special programs for arthritis, burn, and headache patients.

The administrator told us that "we reach out and touch people." Community groups come in, very frequently. "We have dinner meetings with the Lions," he said. "We have kindergarten groups coming through for visits. We greatly try to have people come here when they're well, and thus look at us not just as providers of care but also as an employer and as a resource for the community."

The village of Chelsea had a population of just under four thousand, and the school district between 11,000 and 12,000 students, so that the majority of patients admitted to the hospital came from outside the immediate Chelsea area. "We draw from thirty and more miles," we were told, "and there are a few patients even from Ann Arbor, where the University of Michigan medical school is located."

That psychiatry became early on an established and integral component of the Chelsea hospital the administrator attributed to the fact that "the majority of our physicians are general practitioners who take care, at some level, of psychiatry in their practice while always realizing that they will need additional services. They have felt more comfortable seeing these services in their own community hospital. Probably half of psychiatric patients arrive here via the interaction of the primary care physicians and the psychiatric component."

The psychiatry service was headed medically by two psychiatrists who worked in tandem, Dr. Joseph Meadows Jr. and Dr. Frank Colligan, and the staff included fully trained personnel of other germane disciplines.

Because the hospital had an open staff, any attending physician may admit a patient to the psychiatry service, and follow him. This happened from time to time and evidently had given rise to no notable difficulties or problems. Similarly, members of the courtesy staff may admit and follow psychiatric patients, and occasionally they did so, again, evidently, without difficulties or problems.

Additional to being a readily accessible and competently operated service for those with psychiatric hospitalization need, the unit is unusual and notable for intrahospital relationships. This hospital, among only 116 beds, has, additional to customary surgical and medical wards, the above-mentioned special units. The general wards and the several special units have been developed and fostered into an impressive totality. The psychiatric unit itself seems to be very much a part of the hospital. It operates as an integral component; as a seemingly small—but in reality not small—example, its nurses wear uniforms, and not by chance but as the result of careful deliberation about whether they should; as a larger example, its nurses occasionally are assigned to fill in on other services, and the reverse also occurs.

*   *   *

In the advent from nursing home, the Chelsea facility evolved as planned into a general community hospital, and from 1973 onward was so licensed. (In Michigan, a community hospital is a public hospital owned by a city.) The town of Chelsea had bought the facility from the establishing, and departing, physician. Of the setting of rules and regulations which are reserved to the local authorities, significant input came from the hospital's board of directors. These directors were described to us as "overseers much like any other board of directors," but, it was added, there had developed a tremendous community spirit concerning the emerging hospital, such that "the board may well have had, and still have, input beyond that of other kinds of boards."

The Chelsea area, we were told, "is a very well-informed community," not so distant from the University of Michigan for there not to be some effect. The Chelsea environs have prosperous farms, and, one informant told us, "There's a lot of money here in the rich land." Another told us that it might be more accurate to denote the area "not as one of gentlemen farmers, but of gentlemen who are, on the side, farmers."

The transformation of the facility to a community-owned hospital was well advanced when a six-bed psychiatric unit came into being. The necessary licensure for the original small psychiatric service was readily obtained. When subsequently the psychiatric unit was almost tripled in size, to 16 beds, no new facilities were added. Rather, beds and rooms that had been designed for regular medical patients were simply redesignated psychiatric beds constituting a psychiatric unit.

*   *   *

In those early days, a pattern of psychiatric medical staffing that is now history was unusual enough to warrant mention.

Chelsea Community Hospital

There were at that time two colleague psychiatrists who divided responsibility for the psychiatry service on the basis of alternating weeks. During Week A, psychiatrist A was the physician attending all psychiatric patients. On the alternating week, he was in another part of the country. During Week B, the second psychiatrist served as attending physician for all psychiatric patients; and on his alternating week, he, too, was in another part of the country. How this pattern ever came about we did not explore, but it is notable in the history of the unit for the evident dissatisfaction it engendered in all quarters. It is understatement to say that there was a feeling among the staff bordering on unreality, there was friction seemingly stemming from the arrangement itself, there were resignations of essential trained staff; and all this in the face of a growing psychiatric census that frequently exceeded the authorized number of beds. This unusual pattern of medical management seemed to have become, by the time of our visit, not much more than a disagreeable historic note. But two things were clearly remembered: the growing number of psychiatric admissions indicated an important need to obtain the licensure for a larger unit; and the need to have the medical responsibility for it assigned to regularly available psychiatrists was essential. Both were accomplished.

The new psychiatric director, it was stipulated, was to be on the premises some 48 weeks out of the year. Such a director was recruited, from the medical school in Ann Arbor; and a sense of order was not long in coming. Only about a year later, however, the new director departed to accept a job offer elsewhere.

The psychiatric census by then, under the new 16-bed allocation, averaged about 80 percent—a rate slightly higher than in other departments of the hospital—and the psychiatric unit maintained the staff stabilization that had emerged. In time the unit acquired a half-time and fully trained psychologist, and a considerable allotment of service from the hospital-wide social and occupational therapy services.

*   *   *

Following the departure of the director of psychiatry who had supplanted the original dual directors, Dr. Joseph Meadows entered the picture, and he had been, for several years prior to our visit, a mainstay. He had worked as a general practitioner for some years before he returned to training to complete a residency in psychiatry. Thereafter, he had conducted an outpatient psychiatric practice—a clinic—in Ann Arbor. After almost a score of years in such practice, he came to decide, he told us, that "I had to do something different; I needed some challenge and also more involvement with medical colleagues outside of an office."

It was the aforementioned psychologist from whom Dr. Meadows learned that a chief of psychiatry was being sought at Chelsea. The psychologist had not come originally to Chelsea to work at the community hospital, but at a satellite service of the community mental health center serving that part of Michigan, and operating, some few hours a week, near the facility that was in process of becoming Chelsea Community Hospital. The psychologist arranged to relocate to the hospital since she perceived that the mental health center satellite was expanding in numbers of staff who had less and less training, whereas the psychiatry service of the hospital was growing in ways she found more consistent with her interests and persuasions; for example, the psychiatrist who spent a year as head of the hospital's psychiatry service had introduced a requirement that each inpatient be seen by his therapist—whether that therapist be a psychiatrist or another designated mental health professional assuming the therapeutic responsibility while the psychiatrist was physician of record—on four days a week, and not on four consecutive days. With that psychiatrist departing, Dr. Meadows explored the possibility of arranging to spend part of his time as head of the Chelsea Hospital's psychiatry service, handling administration and planning, involved in coordinating psychiatry with the other departments of the hospital, and supervising staff. It was arranged that the hospital would pay him a salary to take on these activities, based on about ten hours a week; and during some additional hours he was to be attending physician on a fee-for-service basis for some of the psychiatric patients. And beyond this, he would continue to spend about half of his time continuing with the service he had begun and developed in Ann Arbor. It was a conglomeration of activities and settings that he found satisfying.

His later-arrived colleague, Dr. Colligan, also salaried by the hospital for the equivalent of a day a week, was also attending physician for some of the psychiatric inpatients.*

*   *   *

Although a physician must of necessity have the legal and ultimate responsibility for each psychiatric patient, there were

---

*We will omit from this report the substance abuse service, despite the fact that it is situated side by side of the psychiatric service, since it had different and quite separate origins, was run by an almost totally separate staff, and had, evidently by design, little interaction with the psychiatric service. There was between these two units not so much a feeling of competition as of separateness and of separate identities. In the uncertainty of some general hospitals of how to deal simultaneously with substance abuse (particularly alcoholism) patients and "other" psychiatric patients, here was one answer: run collateral services that are essentially separate. That this arrangement might change was suggested by intrahospital discussion that Dr. Meadows would, in no great time, be designated "director of psychiatry" and head up both units, while Dr. Colligan would be designated "director of inpatient psychiatry." This was still under exploration at the time of our visit.

also on the staff three other persons with the designation of therapist—all persons with considerable training. The evident principal reason for this arrangement was to provide for every patient a specified trained, senior staff member who would be engaged in individual interaction beyond what the time allocation of the two psychiatrists permitted. One of these three therapists was the psychologist above described, salaried by the hospital for approximately half time. She devoted her hours at Chelsea for the most part to individual, and sometimes to family, sessions with the patients. Because she spent her time at the hospital exclusively with psychiatric patients, her identity within the hospital was understandably different from that of the other two therapists, who were employed full time by the hospital, in a hospital-wide range of activities with several units (of which, more later). The psychologist spent her other hours in office practice, in Ann Arbor, in collaboration with her husband, also a psychologist. She told us that at Chelsea she "observes" psychodynamic concepts but thinks that such an approach is at odds with the inpatient stay—averaging 18 days. Nonetheless, she said, she tries during her typical four sessions per week with each of the patients assigned to her to "get them to be introspective and to be interpretive, in preparation for discharge."

The two other persons designated as therapists were a nurse with graduate degree and considerable training in psychotherapy, designated a "clinical specialist," deployed to several services of the hospital but spending much of her time in the psychiatry unit; and a psychiatric social worker, who spent the majority of her work week on the psychiatric unit, part of the time doing a variety of things customarily the province of psychiatric social workers, and the rest of her time as therapist of fact for some of the individual inpatients. All three of these so designated therapists seemed to operate with a good deal of au tonomy; the allocation of particular patients among the three seemed to be made informally but at the same time conscientiously. While each patient must of necessity be assigned to one of the physicians, and while medication prescription and supervision must be handled by Drs. Colligan or Meadows or one of the other attendings, this arrangement for additional, specifically designated therapy time was aboveboard, and it seemed to avoid to a large degree the hierarchical competition that can occur in some patterns of psychiatric inpatient staff deployments.

*   *   *

The essence of the treatment program, according to the social worker who was one of the three designated non-physician therapists, is the team approach. "The whole team—psychiatrists, nursing, social work, occupational therapy, recreational therapy—meets weekly, and we discuss all the patients, pooling our ideas consistently, and working together in order to get the same approach." Dr. Colligan told us he sees the team as a vehicle for viewpoints. "As a psychiatrist," he said, "I see and hear things much differently from the way a recreational therapist, an occupational therapist, or a social worker would. We all freely discuss each patient, and everybody helps to make the decisions." Dr. Colligan feels that getting a patient admitted into the psychiatry program is "about a hundred times easier" in the atmosphere of a hospital such as Chelsea. "Patients are admitted mainly for medical problems, and it is much easier to accomplish transfer to the psychiatric service than to attempt to arrange a transfer to a psychiatric service at some other hospital." But significant to the Chelsea mode of operation, he said, "is the likelihood that we admit psychiatric patients who are less sick, because we admit sooner."

Dr. Colligan thinks it is also significant that the hospital's administration is willing to allocate money to pay for part-time medical administration of the psychiatric unit. "Most small hospitals are attuned to voluntary efforts from medical staff as needed. That can make a zoo out of a psychiatric ward. When you have designated directors, identified as setting policy and philosophy, who protect the nurses from any physicians who may give inappropriate orders, then you can have a good staff, because you can run the inpatient psychiatric unit in a sensible and orderly way."

* * *

In addition to the sessions with the psychiatrists, and with the three other of the staff designated as therapists, a reasonable range of activities is offered to the patients.

Transportation is provided one evening a week to take patients swimming at one of the public schools. One afternoon a week patients are taken bowling. The occupational therapist offers on the ward a variety of arts activities and crafts, and she conducts sessions such as "activities of daily living." The hospital's director of volunteers spends some time in the psychiatric service, and she had, at the time of our visit, two volunteers to assist her there, preparing materials for activities and also, notably, spending time individually with any patients confined to bed.

* * *

The psychiatric service seemed fortunate in having a more than usually experienced charge nurse. Following her basic training in nursing she worked at a well-known and well-reputed small private psychiatric hospital in the midwest. After five years there, she returned to school, took an M.S.W., then taught for two years. She then spent more than two years employed as a medical social worker, decided to return to nursing, taught at the University of Michigan for a time, and then, two-and-a-half years before our visit, accepted a job at Chelsea Community Hospital. She found the offer appealing, she told us, because the system was a small one and because her most satisfying prior work had been as a nurse in inpatient psychiatry. She came to Chelsea, however, before a designated psychiatric unit was established and was then the only nurse on the staff who had experience with psychiatric patients. She soon left. When the hospital later both developed a stipulated psychiatric unit and acquired a sole director of psychiatry, she shortly returned, to become the unit's head nurse.

With her combination of varied and extended experience, we sought out her viewpoint on several matters germane to psychiatric units in general hospitals. What difference had it made within the total hospital to have a relatively large psychiatric unit—16 of 116 beds? Some changes in rules had had to be instituted, she answered, and she felt that they were not of major impact. As examples, previously all of the patients of the hospital had been permitted access to their own cars and to the use of the parking lot. Now, no patients were; what had been a quite informal system of passes had been supplanted by a formal system. But she saw such changes as having proved to be appropriate for all patients. "Nobody ever had thought of them before there was a psychiatric unit," she said. She did not think that any patient anywhere in the hospital had lost anything significant specifically because these certain formalities had needed to be introduced.

We asked what she saw as the rationale for having nurses in psychiatry wear uniforms—as in so many general hospital psychiatric units they do not. She attributed the practice at Chelsea to "good planning." She and others had engaged in predicting "some things that would happen, or tend to happen, when the census was high." Embraced in these were her speculation, and that of others, that for all nurses to wear uniforms would obviate separatism among staff members. She added that she feels the nursing role must be the most flexible within a general hospital, and thus the practice of nurses from all Chelsea's services answering call lights or responding to emergency alarms, consistently.

In this psychiatric unit the nurses are not viewed as "doing" therapy or "being" therapists, but as working in the context of a treatment milieu, seeing themselves as being part of the milieu's therapy while maintaining their self-concept as nurses. "I think there is ample integrity in the role of the nurse," she said.

The orientation of nursing staff concerning medication was consistent with that of the other disciplines. She felt that all of the psychiatric staff believe that medicating should be approached conservatively. "We prefer to use all opportunities to work in other ways with patients," she said. This might, we suggested, limit the admission of patients who without medication pose management problems. She replied that the transfer of patients on grounds of their being unmanageable happened less often than once a month. These cases, she generalized, "are almost always flagrantly psychotic people who, not having responded to the treating environment, are consistently unpredictable and create too much stimulus for the ward." Additionally, the limited physical common areas do not provide sufficient physical separation. (This brought us, once again, to the consideration of space limitations likely to result when regular wards are converted to psychiatric wards. Most of the time, the nurse told us, "this is an incipient problem only, and one which we reduce by means of 'expectation.' The expectations of the hospital are made quite clear. Consequently we have had minimal acting out, in part because most of our patients are sufficiently in contact with reality to heed those expectations.'')

For a unit with capacity of 16, her nursing staff seemed adequate. Divided between day and afternoon shifts, there were four (other) full-time registered nurses, two full-time aides, two part-time registered nurses, and two part-time aides, and there were soon to be arriving two more part-time registered nurses. Did she, we asked, in efforts to fill vacancies, search for staff with specific psychiatric experience? ''I like a staff varied in experience and varied in age,'' she told us. ''If I have the luxury to choose, I will choose someone who I think will complement the staff already on hand. Assuming I have the basic complement of experienced people, I look for someone who looks promising in terms of potential, and for appropriateness of personality—this more than experience specific to a psychiatry ward.''

*   *   *

The licensure of the unit allows only voluntary admissions, and of persons who are 18 or older. There is no seclusion room or other security features, and the staffing ratio is not sufficient to allow one-to-one nurse-patient attendance. Consequently, patients not falling within these limits must be transported, sometimes to a private psychiatric hospital in the vicinity, or, particularly when involuntary admission must be arranged, to the state hospital (or, in some cases, involuntary admission can be arranged at the neuropsychiatric institute of the medical school of the University, in Ann Arbor).

These ''exclusionary'' criteria do not, however, involve any great number of potential admissions. The majority of patients are brought through predetermination and/or because it is generally well understood in the vicinity what types of patients are and can be accepted at Chelsea. Exact diagnostic figures for those admitted were not available, but Dr. Meadows estimated that between a third and two-fifths of all patients warrant a diagnosis of psychotic, and most of the rest are "characterologic" or "neurotic." There are few persons presented with senility, these generally coming from their homes—and usually returning to them, after a period of stabilization or respite.

The great majority of admissions, in fact, of whatever diagnosis, return to their families or to an equivalent private living arrangement. Many who have been inpatients are subsequently seen as outpatients, but the hospitalized clients and the majority of outpatients seen privately in the Chelsea area are not appreciably a single track of people; indeed, many of those hospitalized are the outpatients of the area's psychiatrists who specialize in office practice—and there are a number who do—who do not ordinarily follow hospitalized patients but refer such individuals to Dr. Meadows or Dr. Colligan should need manifest for inpatient care.

*　　*　　*

The evidently successful incorporation of psychiatric services within the Chelsea hospital was notable to those who have seen, at the other extreme, considerable "distancing" between "medicine" and "psychiatry." The integration at this hospital was sufficient to lead to considerable pondering of how it came about. Dr. Meadows ventured that it is in part "a prematurely and insufficiently formed idea of 'what psychiatric patients are all about,' and, from that, an inevitable non-accepting attitude toward them." Such patients, he felt, are frequently seen as something different from what community general hospitals exist for. "I am sure," he told us, "that not enough people really have sat down and given the matter intensive or penetrating thought." He felt that some circumstances at Chelsea unarguably predispose an affective unity of identity—the important role that psychiatry should, and did, play with the burn patients, with the advanced arthritic patients, and with the relatives of both; the decision to have a single social service department for the hospital, and a single occupational therapy department flexibly servicing the component units to the extent needed, and adapting their program to make their components suitable for patients in psychiatry; and the practice of having all nurses oriented to a "unihospital" identity. In sum, he felt there was a cultural set that the differences within medicine are secondary to the unity of sensible and adaptable patient care. He felt also that a major factor lay in the experience that both he and Dr. Colligan had had in general practice before they did residencies in psychiatry.

Subsequently

Dr. Meadows advised that by the beginning of 1982 the demand for service had reached the point that there were at times waits of as long as a week, and this despite the fact that he and Dr. Colligan had been joined by a third psychiatrist who divided his time between outpatient and inpatient treatment. The requests for consultation to the other services of the hospital had more than doubled. As for staff, Dr. Meadows had relinquished the post of chief of service in favor of Dr. Colligan; a fourth full-time non-medical therapist had been added; and a trained administrator had been added to concentrate particularly on coordinating the activities of the psychiatric and the substance abuse programs. The inpatients were coming from as far as Ohio and Canada. Dr. Meadows felt the psychiatric unit was providing a particularly useful service for patients with concurrent physical illness, in that "no other hospital in the area wishes to take them, and we have all the facilities and necessary specialties." He added that increased activity on the hospital's campus on the part of the University of Michigan's family practice unit had increased such cases.

Hazleton-Nanticoke Mental Health/ Mental Retardation Unit at Nanticoke State General Hospital Nanticoke, Pennsylvania

I N THE SMALL town of Nanticoke, Pennsylvania, quartered in buildings that are on the grounds of and were once in use by Nanticoke State General Hospital, are located the administrative offices, one of two "regionalized" services, and the sole inpatient service of one of the better and more effective community mental health centers among some dozens which the authors have visited. It is named the Hazleton–Nanticoke Mental Health–Mental Retardation Unit (or center). The inpatient service in particular, but the administrative offices, too, are in Nanticoke rather than in the catchment area's other and larger township of Hazleton because the facilities were available there at start-up time.

The "parent hospital," with its limited but well-defined involvement with the mental health center as a whole and with its inpatient service, is one of nine "state general hospitals" which Pennsylvania built in the 1920's for the specific purpose of serving coal miners who had contracted black lung disease. For the most part, these have been rechanneled into "general community" hospitals, but they are still under the jurisdiction of Pennsylvania's Department of Public Welfare; their funds come from

the state, and their collections go into the state's general reve-
nues. They average about 150 beds and a census of slightly over
sixty percent; only one of the others has a psychiatric service.
There is persistent talk, at varying intensities, of terminating
them and relying on the resources of voluntary general hospitals, but the outcome is not yet clear, at least to the extent that
no definitive ruling has been made nor any specific timetable
adopted.

The 100-bed general hospital at Nanticoke, in addition to
medical/surgical wards, has an intensive care unit, a pediatrics
ward, customary laboratory facilities, and a 24-hour emergency
room. Its board, we were told, had some misgiving about becoming involved with a service for mental patients, in part
because mental health seemed "a strange bird," and in part because the board was concerned that the hospital continue to be
an orderly and neat operation. Said one person long and well
acquainted with the community and the hospital, "There's peace,
but nonetheless an undercurrent, and not all of the medical staff
are comfortable with the mental health operation." But the hospital census had been low, there was unused space, and the
revenue from having it tenanted would help. The hospital could
charge for room and board, remitting a bit—about 20 percent—
to the mental health center, and charging fees for laboratory
work done for mental health patients.

* * *

An important figure, clearly, was the hospital's director of
nursing. She was a member of the mental health center board.
Perhaps more significant, she had worked at the general hospital
for thirty years, had been director of nursing for almost a dozen
years, and, for a time, was interim hospital administrator. She

credits a now departed administrator as having the initial "vision to see that the way to utilize no-longer-needed space was to avail ourselves of the opportunity to collaborate with the community mental health services emerging through federal and state support." She did not lack personal experience, having at one time worked in one of the country's largest mental hospitals. She recalled that the advent of the psychiatric services in two of the Nanticoke buildings so affected nursing staff that "it took about a year to get them settled down." (One local figure suggested that some hospital staff, for some reason, appear to consider the center "a threat to their job security.") The nursing director told us that she realized that the future of the parent hospital was uncertain and that there were differing interests and convictions involved, but she was inclined to think that Nanticoke State General would be viable for the foreseeable future. Dr. Steven Kafrissen, the psychiatrist who is the center's Deputy Director for Clinical Services, is also designated director of the Nanticoke State General Hospital's Division of Psychiatry, and he is the chairman of the hospital's utilization review committee.

* * *

One of the staff characterized Nanticoke as "a little, poor town, not very sophisticated." Family structure remains relatively intact. The catchment area's values impose a high demand for conformity. Attesting to that, we felt, was the fact that on the psychiatric inpatient service, "behavior disordered" teenage patients observed rules and regulations quite well—perhaps because the culture expects "even crazy people" to behave, so that most of them can and do. Mental health center staff dress "like most people," and not idiosyncratically.

In this locality, mental illness still carries considerable stigma; people who have the means are likely to go out-of-area for treatment; and the feeling persists to some extent that mentally ill people get "put away."

Coal mining, once a big industry, was now shrunk to some strip mining, but the amount and variety of manufacturing had grown. Nanticoke's "city" is Wilkes-Barre, some dozen miles away, where there are two general hospitals having psychiatric inpatient services. In drawing catchment area boundaries in Pennsylvania, the rationale for a Hazleton-Nanticoke area appeared mainly to have been that both towns already had outpatient mental health clinics which could be expanded. The catchment area, with a population of 150,000, has only one psychiatrist in private practice, part time, and "miscellaneous other" private practitioners, of no great combined extent for the population size.

Technically, the inpatient unit is part of the general hospital, which bills third parties for psychiatric patients under its provider number. It maintains in its records those of psychiatric patients—and supplemental records are kept in accordance with the mental health center's clinical policies and procedures and the state's regulations.

The center opened in 1972, earlier than had been planned, because Hurricane Agnes had flooded out a nearby center. It now consists of separate Hazleton and Nanticoke units, each providing emergency, intake, day treatment, and outpatient services, plus the single inpatient ward at Nanticoke, and a "transitional living facility," namely a 12-bed halfway house which had opened shortly before our visit. (Additionally, there is a state-operated "domiciliary" program for those who are 18 or older; it serves some with mental illness, some medical cases, and the destitute elderly, placing them into private homes in groups up to three, with placement and monitoring by the Bureau of the Aged.)

The center director since 1973, James Lawlor, is a social worker. There are deputy directors for clinical services, for community services, and for administration. Deputy Director Kafrissen was working at NIMH when he learned, in 1972, that a search was on for a project officer for emergency mental health services being rendered to Hurricane Agnes victims in northeastern Pennsylvania. He took the job and represented NIMH, working with Dr. Edward Hoffman, the local project director, who later became the center's deputy director for community services. They had fifty "paraprofessionals" working with them, visiting flood victims in their homes, helping them to get loans, and giving them counsel intended to help them tolerate and deal with the shock of the losses dealt them. When that emergency effort was nearing its end, Kafrissen learned that the mental health center at Nanticoke might need medical staff, surveyed the situation, and applied. He had long been interested in community psychiatry, "not in the sense of ministering to the problems of society or of dissatisfactions with life, but in the sense of how to provide local treatment to disturbed people." He had been in his job at Nanticoke for six years when we talked with him. He liked the fact that his work had variety, and he liked the life style of the locality and "would not want to go back to the big-city rat race." One source of variety was his work each week with 25 adolescent boys in a children's home in Hazleton; he also did the psychiatric portion of a project providing aftercare services for 120 mental patients. But he sometimes felt isolated and relied on opportunities to attend conferences and workshops as a means of access to cultural and collegial stimulation.

The only other psychiatrist in the center serves as "fill-in"

for the inpatient unit and takes his turn on after-hours emergency calls but mainly provides the medical service for the various parts of the Hazleton and Nanticoke "community" units,
whose directors work with him. This doctor, Robert F. Babskie,
had spent 12 years in general practice, then did a residency in
psychiatry, partly at a state hospital. After undergoing some sur-
gery that somewhat reduced his mobility, he became superinten-
dent of the Retreat State Hospital, a few miles from Nanticoke,
then worked for a time for the state mental health office, and in
time came to the Hazleton-Nanticoke center, where he is "very,
very happy." He said psychiatrists have to work comparatively
hard in this program, and it has been difficult to attract an additional one who is qualified.

*　　*　　*

The inpatient unit, which like all components of the center
hires its own personnel, is housed on the second floor of what
was the dormitory for nursing students when the hospital had a
nursing school. It can accommodate 18 patients, all in semiprivate rooms, each with its own bath. At one end is a small room
used for change-of-shift and other staff meetings; in the center,
and open to the corridor, is a reasonably nice patient lounge of
adequate size and with kitchen equipment. The nursing station
is unsatisfactorily but necessarily located in a room that allows
no observation of patients. Nonetheless, the unit is unlocked,
albeit with the precaution of "buzzered" doors, which sound a
loud alert in the event of an unauthorized exit. The unit is modest, clean, and pleasant. There are laundry facilities for patient
use, and there is an area of adequate size for physical exams
and cardiopulmonary resuscitation. There is a pay telephone which
patients may make reasonable use of from about 7:00 a.m. to
11:00 p.m. One level lower, on the ground floor, are some of-

fices and a fairly large room variously used for day-patient activities (sometimes attended by some of the inpatients), for family-patient-staff joint sessions, and court hearings for involuntarily committed patients.

The unit has registered nurses on duty at all times; there are seven of them, plus two licensed practical nurses and seven mental health workers at Grades I, II, and III according to education and experience. There are at least one man and one woman on every shift. The unit has a "co-ordinator" who "birddogs" patient plans, a caseworker, who spends much of her time with the patients' relatives, and an activity therapist— a young Juilliard graduate who seemed to us perhaps as ingenious, imaginative, and energetic—and self-taught—as any of numerous activity therapists we have seen in action. He does seven groups per week, "trying to use activities as a springboard to get into problems in an unthreatening way, hoping to help people loosen up so that they can discuss things more easily."

The head nurse had "come home" after working elsewhere; although she had no mental health experience, she applied for this job because nursing jobs thereabouts were scarce. She evidently had adapted readily and well, but she found the rate of rehospitalization "disappointing," and occasionally she—like others of the staff—was perturbed by a rebellious teenage patient.

Other staff, not to be overlooked since they have important roles, are a doctoral psychologist, Joseph Romesser, with the title of Residential Services Unit Director, who among other things heads the daily morning and change-of-shift staff meetings, and Richard Walsh, a social worker who, as deputy to Dr. Kafrissen, is Clinical Services Coordinator, charged with "implementing and reviewing" all clinical (more precisely residential) policies and procedures; he had been for a time director of the Hazleton unit.

Ratio of staff to patient at full inpatient census is approximately one-to-one. There seemed to be a consensus that the staffing was adequate and appropriate.

*   *   *

Getting in. Any self-presenting or escorted applicant starts at the Hazleton or the Nanticoke unit, except after hours. On evenings and weekends, in addition to a ''sleep-in'' emergency worker, a psychiatrist and an experienced and trained crisis worker are ''beeper equipped.'' (On the Saturday prior to our visit, the emergency worker on call had more than thirty calls, some involving child welfare, some being domestic squabbles in which the police had become involved. The emergency beeper seemed much like an all-purpose hotline.) If a potential case is presented and admission seems indicated, the psychiatrist comes in person to handle the admission, declining to admit via telephone authorization. Some prospects for admission seem to suggest the need for a period of observation, so they are medicated and ''sat with.'' Persons who seem to be merely vagrant are put up at a motel. The police or relatives can bring in anyone for evaluation, or by petition, on the grounds that the individual is seriously emotionally disabled, meaning, in theory, that there seems reason to think that if he is not given care within thirty days he may die. In many of the small communities in the catchment area, as it happens, the police are acquainted with most residents and can readily get their cooperation.

A ''personal profile'' is done for each new inpatient, consisting of his family tree, going back two generations and indicating those ancestors with a history of mental illness, alcoholism, and suicide, attempted or accomplished, and identifying significant others, whether related or not, who may be available to support the patient in one or more ways. Within 24 hours of admission, a physical examination is done by a physician employed by the mental health center from the Nanticoke Hospital staff.

* * *

The patients. At the time of our visit, the census was high, but almost half of the patients were from a neighboring center which has arranged to send its "overload" to Nanticoke. A Nanticoke psychiatrist inventoried permissable grounds for hospitalization as *a*) "lethality," *b*) the need to detach the patient temporarily from a pathological support system showing promise that it can be modified, or *c*) the need for heavy medication.

The patient group when we visited was diverse, ranging in age from adolescent to elderly and having some cases each of schizophrenia and serious depression, some sociopathic younger patients, and some patients with histories of extensive heavy drinking. Those whose presenting problem is alcohol must need "more than" detoxification. There have been no "drugged out" prospective patients, but there have been addicted patients who, while on the unit, have been "tapered off." With many patients, relatively heavy doses of medication are used initially; electroshock is not used at all. Leather restraints are available but rarely used, and then only with frequent observation.

The patients have a relatively full program. Each morning the staff gathers for a "precommunity meeting" to consider passes, privileges, discharges, and the like, following which there is a "patient community meeting." The patients are "self-governed," electing officers each week, deciding on passes, and setting or revoking other privileges on the basis of presence or absence of disruptiveness, bizarre thinking, ability to exercise care, and so on—but the staff may veto privileges if they appear to have been misdealt. (Privilege levels are *a*) to leave the unit or the building when accompanied by a staff member, *b*) to leave the unit but not the building with a fellow patient having the same privilege, and *c*) to leave the unit, but not the building, alone.) After lunch there is another group session, which may consist of a discussion, sometimes with the men and the women meeting separately, a walk, or an activity. The center has two vans that are used to take patients shopping, bowling, or to the movies. Visiting hours are from four to eight p.m. (longer on Saturdays and Sundays), and most patients have concerned relatives who come and "are a big part of the therapy." (Patients frequently have passes to spend weekend days at home.) At eight o'clock comes the final patient group of the day, largely to discuss the next day's plans.

The patient group meetings on which we sat in were impressive; all patients attended, and there was an agenda. Four staff were present, one to take notes. At one meeting in particular, there seemed an air of apathy, perhaps denoting the severity of pathology; at this meeting, a young hallucinated male wanted increased privileges, which the patients were almost casually inclined to grant, so that the staff had to extend itself via comments clarifying the patient's situation and thus redirecting the group's attitude. At another, led by the activity therapist, patients sat in a circle, while one, in the center, was "given the power," obligating him to do at least something. One directed the group to sing, another told them to switch seats, and one directed a 16-year-old to kiss an elderly woman, who then "perked up" noticeably. At the end of the session, the activity therapist made observations to the patients about their leadership styles—how commanding had worked for some, explaining for others, how some quiet patients became more verbal. It seemed an example of "utilizing dynamic interaction in the here and now." The change-of-shift staff meeting was similarly impressive—sensible and thorough. The staff understands disruptive behavior, the impact on patient of transfer from one facility to another, and the like. They were deeply distressed that the transfer schedule for one young patient had been messed up by another agency, but despite their concern for him and their supposition that he might elope, they worked instead to rearrange and rectify the timing rather than even suggest that he be "respited" via extending his hospitalization. This suggested to us a high sense of responsibility in approving hospital stay only on grounds of clear, specific need.

The average length of stay is about 18 days—slightly longer than the national average for general hospital psychiatric units. Perhaps inevitably one bright and young staff member with some graduate training lamented the "too short" stay and was convinced that it explained the "high" readmission rate. We heard statements to this effect frequently during this study. It seems evident that there is a faith that if one keeps a patient 16 days instead of eight, or thirty days instead of 15, he or she will be likely to get "more well" and to stay that way much longer, even though there are no definitive data to substantiate this viewpoint. It seems difficult for some mental health practitioners to accept that some forms of mental illness, like a number of "purely physical" illnesses, are cyclic, phasic, and/or frequently relapsing or recurrent. Since for many patients hospitalization is not a pleasure, it could be equally maintained that, in a year, two inpatient stays of ten days may have advantages over a single stay of a month.

*   *   *

Inservice training. The offerings were appropriately varied and frequent. In a nine-month period shortly before our visit, there were 134 staff enrollments in courses which typically meet once a week, for an hour and a half, for six weeks. Subjects included: diagnosis, assessment, and psychopharmacology, taught by a psychiatrist; interviewing techniques, taught by a social worker; family therapy, taught by a psychologist; cardiopulmonary resuscitation, taught by an American Heart Association person; plus courses on group therapy, values clarification, and movement therapy. Other courses soon to be offered were on "burn out," relaxation therapy techniques, mental health concepts and practice, and "the environment of the aged."

Miscellany and synopsis. This center is impressive, perhaps particularly to those who have seen a variety of centers. A few years ago about 150 people per year went from this catchment area into the state hospital; while it is within a half hour of the center, its admissions from the catchment are now only about one per month—even though judges occasionally order patients directly there for security reasons, since the center has no security room. When the state hospital is discharging a patient, it makes a specific appointment for him with the center, and if the patient does not keep it, a center staff member goes to the patient's home. Some of the residents of the still-new halfway house were already spending their days back at their jobs.

As a means of "quality assurance review," the formulated inpatient process includes initial assessment, including mental status examination, medical history, assessment of suicide potential, and social history; a preliminary treatment plan formulated within 24 hours with clearly defined goals, indication of services needed, and statement of contributions needed from other agencies; progress notes indicating changes in level of function and provision for continuity of care and follow-up, an account of problems that have arisen, and emerging indications for change in treatment plan; then, on release, a written statement of final diagnostic impression, prognosis, medication schedule, and recommendations to client for further treatment.

Treatment seems to be well integrated. Patients can move easily between and among elements—the emergency service, outpatient appointments, day treatment, hospitalization, and the halfway house. There seems little concern about territoriality, little "dumping," and much common sense. The inpatient unit impresses one as having a "community-milieu approach" akin to that formulated by Maxwell Jones. (Anent one comment about "shortness" of stay, putatively a sixty-day stay is possible, since in Pennsylvania Medicaid permits that length of psychiatric hospitalization in a general hospital.) One local official felt the center "had promised more than it could deliver"; another wished that general practice physicians would make a better effort to learn about psychotropic medication use and drug interactions. As for the authors, we felt there was an unusually competent and devoted staff and that Dr. Kafrissen was a remarkable instance of simultaneous idealism and practicality.

Subsequently

The state mental hospital nearby (Retreat) was closed in 1980 because of consolidation by the state. Since then, patients in need of longer-term care, or a more secure setting, must go to a state hospital fifty miles away.

The future of Nanticoke State General Hospital was by mid-1982 unclear.

The number of private psychiatric beds had increased within

the county, with 18 opened at a new 250-bed medical center just outside Wilkes-Barre.

There had also been changes within the Hazleton-Nanticoke Mental Health/Mental Retardation Center, with three full-time psychiatrists including one each in the Hazleton and Nanticoke units, the other continuing as medical director of the inpatient service and providing clinical and administrative leadership for the operations of the center.

Services had been expanded or modified. The federal staffing grant ended. The halfway house was turned over to a non-profit agency (Step-by-Step, Inc.) which was able to decrease operating costs and still provide a locally based transitional living facility. A new children's service, known as SCAN, was started.

The director of nursing at Nanticoke State General Hospital became president of the board of the center.

The physical structure of the inpatient service had been improved, with a more conventional nursing station, more accessible and allowing full monitoring of all patient rooms. The community area, now enclosed, contained more agitated or confused patients, to beneficial effect.

The "openness" of the unit was modified with the locking of the rear door, since staff were not adequately able to monitor patients with that door unlocked. The front door and elevator, easily watched, still provided easy access.

Emergency patients brought for mental health evaluations were seen, after hours, in Nanticoke Hospital's emergency room. If admission was indicated, transfer to the inpatient unit was arranged, and the psychiatrist on call contacted for orders.

There was both a full-time and a half-time caseworker assigned to the inpatient service, and a half-time activities specialist (who replaced the music therapist).

Patients frequently started attending one of the five partial hospitalization programs on a "transitional basis" while still inpatients.

Nurses were now all registered nurses, even though R.N. recruitment and retention was a major problem. Salaries were being increased, including a significant shift differential.